MAKING A DIFFERENCE

WAYS TO MAGNIFY ABUNDANCE, VITALITY & FREEDOM IN YOUR LIFE

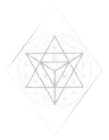

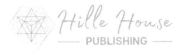

Hille House
PUBLISHING

Editing: Ruth Fae
Formatting: Megan Falzarano
Book Cover Design: Dragoslav Andjelkovic

Disclaimer:
The authors in this book do not dispense medical advice or prescribe the use of any technique as a form of treatment for physical, emotional, or medical problems without the advice of a physician, either directly or indirectly. The intent of the authors is only to offer information of general nature to help you on your quest for emotional, physical, and spiritual well-being. In the event the readers use any of the information in this book for themselves, the authors and the publisher assume no responsibility for their actions.

CONTENTS

INTRODUCTION

Dear Reader,

I am so glad that you are holding this book in your hands. I honour you for taking this step. We worked very hard to bring every little letter to you and there is a reason. In fact, there are three reasons: abundance, vitality and freedom, because we want you to walk away with more of them.

Why these three qualities?

For me, these three areas are the most important for realising potential, happiness, and joy because, as we have freedom from patterns of the past, we can enter into more meaningful relationships with ourselves and others. It's about being conscious of the "Internal Scripts" (as you can read in my chapter) and changing any that no longer serve you.

By releasing the patterns/scripts around abundance and scarcity we can breathe into and access deeper levels of inner peace, and from that place can make an even greater difference in the world as we are not so preoccupied with our own survival. From that place of inner safety, I have felt more confident in "poking the bear," in seeking to change the status quo for the better for all.

Our mental health or vitality features in many of the chapters, how the authors have Made A Difference (M.A.D.) in their own lives, and now in the lives of others through their work.

How did the concept of M.A.D. come to be so meaningful to me?

In 2022 our business, Your Words Have Power, was shortlisted for the ROAR Business Awards (Australian accolade) for the MAD category. Initially, I felt ambivalent about the acronym, and as I sat with it, I realised it crystalised the concept of what I had been doing all my life without putting a name to it. It ignited the spark to intentionally structure my work around this and thus the theme of this book was kindled.

I have been part of another multi-author book and the very process of writing a part of my story saw a massive growth in me. We had a book reading and signing here in Perth and I offered my services to my fellow authors to coach them to read from their chapter to an audience.

I realised this is not an innate skill, so I wanted to offer my concept "From Page to Stage" to my fellow authors in that book. Furthermore, I wanted to extend the opportunity and offer it to authors in a new volume. Other people who share my MAD vision could not only share their wisdom on paper, they could begin/build a speaking career from their book too.

We have tales set in Australia, Canada, Cambodia, New Zealand, Singapore, and the USA. Our authors take you on journeys that will leave you on the edge of your seat with all the plot twists that can happen in life: business, childhood, parenting, mental health, and adulthood.

Our Authors come from diverse backgrounds. All share part of their life story, and the wisdom and insights gained from those experiences in their own lives. From reading by lamplight in rural Cambodia to being part of a global organisation; from suicidal to empowering coach, we invite you to consider how that wisdom can be used to Make A Difference in your own life and also in the lives of others.

Dive into the chapters; recognise where those themes are relevant to you. Ignite that fire within you so that you, too, can Make A Difference!

Let the transformation begin!

Wendy Corner
Lead Author

WENDY CORNER

THE UNINTENTIONAL ENTREPRENEUR

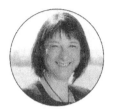

*I*ve been MAD all my life! Not always intentionally, I admit.

Intention is a powerful thing, but here's the rub. You can set your intention to, well, intentionally Make A Difference, know the actions you intend to take to make that difference and still not get the outcome you intended! Does that sound familiar?

Recently I found myself watching a seminar that promised to be, "the last training I would ever need" in the self-development sphere. It was a "Revolutionary New Breakthrough." I found myself saying out loud, "Yep! I know all that. Nothing new here." This was quickly followed by that voice in my head saying, "So why haven't you done anything with that info?" I recognised that Inner Voice, except this wasn't that familiar, snidey critical voice. This was the gentle voice of my Guidance inviting me to delve deeper and ask myself from a place of love, "Why "haven't" you done what you know to be effective?" The invitation was to shine the spotlight on my Internal Scripts.

WHAT DO I MEAN BY INTERNAL SCRIPTS?

Scripts are the words we say to ourselves, especially when no one is watching. Some call them *Limiting Beliefs* and, doubtless, some truly are constricting, limiting, even paralysing. And yet some are empowering, expansive and purposeful. Sometimes these Scripts can be at a conscious level and all-too-often they are at an unconscious level as they have been so well rehearsed that they become our default mode.

I liken them to procedural memory. Remember the first time you tried to tie your shoelaces, or balanced on your bike without your trainer wheels, or started learning to drive? All took intention. All took focus. All took practice until they became procedural memory. Now you no longer have to think consciously or intentionally through every step of the sequence, right? Like the autopilot has been switched on.

So it is with your Scripts. They are forged, very often, at a young age. This usually occurs up to the age of seven, when your brain is in that gorgeous, gummy, totally "plastic" stage of development. (There's a shed load of science regarding the frequency of brain waves, critical thinking and the like, which I'm happy to geek out about with you in a different arena!) These early Scripts came about at a time in life when we were not able to question them. They could be created by what we heard directed to us. For example, "Shut up! Be quiet!" translated into the Script to keep quiet and not speak your truth. Your opinion doesn't matter.

Have you ever found yourself saying those same words, with this addition, "Who wants to listen to you anyway?" Sometimes you can distinctly "hear" the voice and recognise the person who gave you this Script—a critical parent/teacher. As a child, I was removed from class for talking. Those who know me will say that I'm not often lost for words. Yet I never told my parents about this, *ever!*

If you can identify those voices, those Scripts, you can acknowledge that that is someone else's opinion and not your own, even if you unwittingly adopted it. Some of these Scripts, however, are buried deep inside your unconscious and the memories associated with them may have been buried too. That's not to say that, just because you are not conscious of them, they are not having a powerful impact on your life at an unconscious, an unintentional, level.

This is the story of the "Unintentional Entrepreneur" and how my Scripts have impacted this journey. I'm going to explore the five most significant Scripts I have uncovered to date. Some have been empowering so I have kept those. Some were certainly not serving me, particularly as an entrepreneur, and so with the awareness came the choice to flip them to Scripts that are empowering. Here, I share incidents in my life that have uncovered the Scripts and at the end of the chapter, I list the five empowering Scripts I now play. *I wonder if they resonate with the Scripts you are playing at the unconscious level?* We make decisions, intentionally or otherwise, about how we are going to react or respond (knee-jerk or deliberately thought through).

What do I mean by that? Let me take you back to a pivotal moment in my early life.

It's 1968, an era when parents were banned from staying in hospital with their children. It's at this time that an almost three-year-old required surgery and her whole world fell apart. As the double doors closed with Mam on one side and me on the other, screaming for her, she was unable to come to my aid. When you are two, your world revolves around you, right? If things don't happen the way you expect or want them to, you have something to say/scream/jump and down about, right? That's developmentally appropriate!

SIGNIFICANT SCRIPT #1: MY VOICE DOESN'T MATTER

Wee Wendy decided that, "My voice doesn't matter! Everybody else's voice does!" At that point, I buried that memory deep in my subconscious and I had no concept of how that internal script would unintentionally play out in my life.

There were various times I made a conscious choice in regard to this Script.

I intended to Make A Difference by supporting someone else to shine by not putting myself forward for the "leading lady" role in our primary school film, even although it meant giving up on the chance to kiss Jimmy Holloway, the boy I had a crush on. I let my friend take the role and I was assigned "Continuity Mistress" instead. I intentionally held back because of my unintentional Internal Script - my voice didn't matter and hers did.

3

However, I was able to Make A Difference in her life, and the quality of the film as I was *brill-i-ant* at spotting when something was different from the last take/scene.

Fast forward a few years to when I am considering career choices.

I always wanted to do something medical when it came to, "what I wanted to be when I grew up." Fascinated by the human body, being a doctor was the obvious choice, however that required Maths, Physics and Chemistry at A-Level (major exams in the UK) to qualify entry into Medical School. I didn't stand a chance! Two of the three subjects were so out of reach because I simply didn't understand them. I was far more Humanities-based and loved language so instead, I took Latin at A-Level. Unlike my friends who had clear career goals, my A-Level choices did not take me intentionally towards a particular subject to study at Uni or an obvious career. Music, Latin, and Religious Studies—with that combo, was I going to be a Nun?

So, having ruled out medicine, I looked at the Allied Health Professions (AHP). Physio? I wasn't enough of a bully and in my experience, Physios had to be bullies to get folks to do what hurt. Occupational Therapist? Nope! Baskets really didn't float my boat. (Horrible stereotype which I later apologised to my OT colleagues for.) I was drawing a blank as I sat in the canteen in the Sixth Form Centre until one of my friends handed me a university prospectus and asked if I'd seen Speech Therapy. She knew I loved language and was always slipping into one accent or another. I looked at the Prospectus and off went a lightbulb—I could do something vaguely medical *and* combine that with my love of words, and language, and Make A Difference to people! This was certainly an intentional choice!

Except that I was rejected by all the universities that I applied for. With all my friends successfully going to Uni, I was left behind, so I decided to do an extra A-level and re-apply the following year. My school was so helpful, and the timetable was engineered so that I could attend classes for both Year Eleven and Twelve. The Head of Biology was a wonderfully supportive woman, as was the Head of Sixth Form. I intentionally worked my butt off that year and squeezed a two-year course into one.

And still, I was rejected by all the universities I applied to! By this point, I'll admit, I was pretty demoralised. One of my friends who offered a supportive ear commented that she didn't know how I was keeping my pecker up. In response, I came out with this statement, "He who perpetually lives under the surface will sooner or later drown!" Where on earth did that little profound gem come from?

SIGNIFICANT SCRIPT #2: YOUR MIND CREATES YOUR REALITY

Some twenty-five years later, when doing a Tony Robbins course, I learned that I was creating my own reality based on what I was focusing on. (That enabled me to put words to this Script!) If you're thinking about red cars as you are driving, you'll see lots of them, more than normal—because that's what you're focusing on. I was in my late thirties before I heard this, and it only really made sense ten years later!

Back to the story. Now, what was I going to do?

I knew in my heart of hearts that I was going to be a "Speechie" and train in London but I had no idea how this was going to happen. Again, a friend looking through a prospectus of courses in AHP asked if I had come across the *School for the Study of Disorders of Human Communication*. What a mouthful! I applied on "Clearing," the "last chance" way in after all the exam results are in and the Universities know how many places they have, based on how many students have achieved the required grades. I had an offer, which I didn't meet—I needed a B-grade and got a C-grade. The day the results came out (a Thursday), I phoned the Department Head who said he'd think about it over the weekend. That was the longest weekend of my life!

On Monday when I phoned, he said, "I think you're alright!" What on earth did that mean? I had to intentionally ask him for clarity and so with that "yes," my journey of Making A Difference in the lives of people with communication problems began.

SIGNIFICANT SCRIPT #3: TRUST YOUR GUIDANCE, NO MATTER WHAT THE CIRCUMSTANCES LOOK LIKE!

Over the course of almost thirty years of clinical practice, I worked with approximately five thousand individuals alongside their respective ecosystems—family, school/work/carers. I intentionally set out to impact their ability to communicate successfully because their voice mattered! (#1) I worked primarily with adults (some children at first) with voice problems, intellectual disability, Autistic Spectrum Disorder, challenging behaviour, and some forensic work too. Always, my intention was to Make A Difference—and I did!

During this time, I was employed by the National Health Service (NHS) in the UK. I've migrated twice now, the first was from England to Scotland so that we could have a change in pace of life as my husband was mentally unwell. We intended to Make A Difference to his well-being. When he died very suddenly fifteen years later, I was advised not to make any life-changing decisions for at least six months until I had settled into a new routine.

Wise words indeed, as I unintentionally found myself facing an identity shift. No longer a wife and carer. No longer Making A Difference in Geoff's life and, after twenty years of marriage, that took some time to adjust to. During our marriage, I had made assumptions. A big one was that we were going to have a family and, ten years into the marriage when I finally plucked up the courage to raise the topic, I was clearly told there was never any intention to have children, at least not from his perspective! (#1 is why it took that long to mention it.)

SIGNIFICANT SCRIPT #4: OTHER PEOPLE ARE MORE IMPORTANT THAN I AM

Three years later I came on a trip to Australia. It was the last thing I was to do for Geoff: to visit his cousin and aunt in the Blue Mountains. This was the journey we always intended to take together, however as he was mentally unwell, he was not able to travel such long distances.

I adored Australia, and whilst appreciating that living and working somewhere is not the same as enjoying a holiday, I still *knew* I was now being called to make a permanent move to Oz. Just as I knew about doing my Speech Therapy study in London despite all the visible signs saying otherwise, I knew that I was to get a job as a Speechie in Australia. (#3) In order to be ready to go when I got the job, I felt led by God to leave my senior role as a Specialist Speechie, and pack up my belongings (i.e., declutter from the "stuff" I had accumulated from losing my father-in-law, mother-in-law, brother-in-law, and husband over ten years).

I intended to make a fresh start in Australia with minimal material stuff coming with me. You remember how my journey to study Speech Therapy didn't go smoothly? Well, guess what? Neither did my journey to Australia!

I left the NHS at the end of 2012 and didn't secure a job until the end of September. Then came the wait for the visa, except I "knew" I would get the visa so my container of belongings left for Australia before my visa actually came through. What on earth was I thinking?

It made no sense, yet I knew in my heart of hearts that's where I was headed! (#3)

All went well with the job to start with as I was granted a sponsored working visa and, ultimately, my permanent residency. I brought some fresh ideas with me and instigated new ways of working, however, I then discovered something had changed.

There was a misunderstanding and they decided to "let me go." I could have challenged the decision however I decided not to. (#4) I am eternally grateful that they paid for the visas that enabled me to come and stay in Australia. The problem was that my visa was attached to that job. I had another fifteen months to work for them and I couldn't work for another firm or I would face deportation. The Immigration Department wouldn't give me a definitive answer regarding leave to stay in the country, and I wonder if they turned a blind eye? So for fifteen months, I survived on my savings and intentionally used my time productively to qualify as a life coach. (#3)

So here I am after twenty-eight years with a steady income in the corporate world, now faced with being an entrepreneur. Having served my time in limbo, I was free to work again, yet I wouldn't be able to get a job as a Speechie in Perth. It's a small city, and people talk. With a question mark over why I left the company (due to a "misunderstanding") and no reference, I was pushed into the entrepreneurial world. (#1 and #4)

I did not *intend* to be a businesswoman! I had no role models in my close family as both my parents were employed. One uncle, who ran his own Insurance Broking business, always seemed to complain about how much work he had to do without actually getting on with anything. (Or that's what it looked like to the know-it-all teenager who observed him.) (#2 I had no role models and focused on that, and the belief that it was "hard work.")

So, what did it look like, feel like, to be an entrepreneur? That wasn't my plan! My intention was to be a lifelong Speechie where my "leads" came in the form of a waiting list of clients—there had been no need to go out "prospecting." I didn't even understand what prospecting meant. In the NHS, all health care is free at the point of delivery—taxes pay for that. In the company I worked for in Australia, there was a finance department that dealt with the invoicing, another area I had no notion about. And so, Script #5 revealed itself.

SIGNIFICANT SCRIPT #5: I'M NO GOOD WITH NUMBERS

Remember I said that Maths was one of those A-level subjects I couldn't grasp? Yep! Not a great script to run when you are a Business Owner. I had no idea how to deal with revenue, expenses, proposals, or networking. In reality, networking wasn't so much of a stretch as I'm a great people-person. The challenge lay in doing so strategically and systematically. Learning to have an overview, "working *on* my business, not simply *in* my business." This entrepreneurial journey certainly was taking me into unknown territory with a new language and new skills to develop. Without a doubt, the most challenging of personal development journeys as any business cannot outgrow the owner.

Oh me! Talk about stretching out of the familiar! Was this why I came to Australia? To be a businesswoman? How was I going to Make A Difference?

I tried a few niches and, having been head-hunted by the TEDx Team at the University of Western Australia, I had another lightbulb moment— I could become a Speaker Coach! I could combine my experience as a Speechie with voice clients and dust off the system I worked on all those years previously (without it intentionally being a "system"), as well as combining the linguistics, pragmatics, phonetics (all the juicy technical stuff), and the fine degree of non-verbal skills gained working with folks whose verbal skills were limited.

I was back! Making A Difference, intentionally, to the speakers I worked with.

Then the coach who had helped me uncover that script that, "everybody else's voice mattered" challenged me to take out the word "else" and embody, "everybody's voice matters—including mine," and to lead by example! In the time I have worked with her, these five scripts have come to light and, where necessary, have been amended to positively and intentionally serve me!

#1 Everybody's voice matters.

#2 Your mind creates your reality.

#3 Trust your guidance, no matter what the circumstances look like! God sees the big picture; I can only see one metre/three feet in front of me.

#4 I am just as important as everyone else. My business cannot grow beyond my level of self-belief.

#5 Numbers are my friend. They take the emotion out of my business as they are objective.

I may have fallen into being the "Unintentional Entrepreneur," however, now I intentionally Make A Difference not simply to that one individual and their ecosystem of maybe twenty significant others. I could, can, and do Make A Difference to the lives of many, many more. The speakers I work with are impacting hearts and minds from the stage (and now the page too, as I work with the authors in this book and further volumes). *Plus*, as I speak from stage about the *Power of Words* to create impact, to Make A Difference in the lives of all who hear your words (starting with you and every cell in your body responding to those Scripts), the impact is magnified!

I work with powerful speakers who want to see real change in the world. They are not content to settle for the status quo. They have a fire in their belly that requires articulating to the right audience in a way that pokes the bear *and* opens up dialogue. They know that change can only be effective if it is approached from both ends—policy makers and grassroots momentum—and they have the courage to lead the charge!

What a privilege it is to impact hearts and minds as I intentionally *Make A Difference* as an entrepreneur.

ABOUT THE AUTHOR

WENDY CORNER

Wendy Corner is the Quirky Speaker Coach, Bestselling Author, Speaker, and Founder and Creator of Your Words Have Power. She works with global change makers and visionaries who are Making A Difference - speakers on a mission to get their message out to the right audiences.

She and her team work with you to find the best platforms for your message, written and oral, so you can "poke the bear," and achieve that radical new vision from the grass roots up *and* the top down!

Originally from Scotland, Wendy is now based in Perth, Western Australia and has been a TEDx speaker coach at the University of Western Australia since 2018.

With a background as a Speech Pathologist for almost thirty years, Wendy uses a blend of her clinical work, quantum physics, and Internal Scripts in her proprietary framework to support speakers to communicate using body, mind, and spirit to connect at a deep level... to make a Bigger Difference with their audience.

Wendy is committed to MAD (Making A Difference)!

CONNECT WITH WENDY HERE:

Website: https://www.ywhp.events

Free Gift: https://path.ywhp.events/Essential-Speakers-Toolkit

For all socials: https://linktr.ee/commcoach

LIVE LIFE BY DESIGN, NOT DEFAULT

HOW TO ESCAPE STANDARDISED SUCCESS

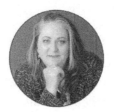

*Y*our life doesn't have to suck. It doesn't have to feel hard, and it doesn't have to feel like you're pushing uphill all the time. Being dissatisfied with the world you have created does not need to be a life sentence; it is absolutely possible to change. But before you can make any changes stick, it's essential to know what you want instead. To be able to set effective goals and have a fighting chance at achieving them, having a clearly defined dream to work towards is pivotal. Without it, it's too easy to fall back into your old paradigms.

But what is it you want instead? What do you dream of? If I asked you to talk me through exactly how you want to live your life, rather than the way you do now, could you describe that to me with absolute clarity?

Many people have fallen into living the life somebody else has wanted for them, or one that has been expected of them, or even living as an extension of their partner's life. Because their world is not entirely of their choosing, dissatisfaction creeps in, closely followed by resentment, anger, and sometimes, depression. And while living a life of "less than" is the current "normal" with most of the people I talk to, I am absolutely not ok with that!

When did it become "normal" to accept a life of less than you deserve?

Why has it become normal? At what point did each of us give up on the dreams we were so passionate about in our younger days to accept the mediocrity of a life lived by default?

Can you pinpoint when you gave up on your dreams? Or was it more like a gradual acceptance of a life defined by the box of your current income, the norms of where you lived and the social group you were part of?

Complacency can creep into our lives like an insidious growth, slowly sucking all the joy and fulfillment from our lives. It played a huge role for me in ending up in a place where I didn't love my life. And it took a few really big shoves from the Universe for me to create a fundamental change in my world, so I could create the life I dreamed of and designed. We all have a different definition of what our "Dream Life" looks like. The standardised version of success is not fulfilling to so many who are trapped living life by default. My mission is to change this, to help people create and live the life they design.

Let me backtrack before I go too much further, to give you more context to this story—my story. In sharing, I want to give you a better understanding of how I came to live the life I have designed, and how this now mirrors the work I do with my clients.

FOUNDATIONS AND FAMILY

I grew up on a cattle property in Queensland, Australia. We were a fairly average family with me the middle child of three, an only daughter with two brothers. Our mother was the stay-at-home parent who took care of the bookwork, fielded phone calls for the business, ran our home, and was very active in roles in the local community. She was always busy but most of her work went unrecognised, and in general, was undervalued, which was also quite normal in my recollection of life as a kid. Dad was, and still is, a grazier. The family farm revolves around the breeding of cattle, which has been my Dad's passion his whole life.

The "men's work" in our family and business, according to my perception then, was "most important." The "men's work" was the outside work, and the outside work was what generated income, so that was far more important than the "inside work" or "women's work." By default, this made the men more important than the women. Rightly or wrongly, this was my take on the dynamic at home when I was a child. But as a strong, intelligent and capable human who happened to be female, I was not happy to accept that status quo! So I did what I could to be as useful as the men and work with them. When my physical strength couldn't match theirs, I did the work that required more dexterity, like taking care of bookwork with my neater handwriting, and vaccinating the cattle while in the crush.

Whenever there was stockwork to be done on the property, all three kids were there with Dad on horseback, working the whole day, helping within the family business. Payment for this work came in the form of choosing a heifer (female) calf at the end of the year to extend our personal herd. These cattle were managed alongside the main herd and treated the same way, which taught us so much about business. Ideas like living the repercussions of our choices, delayed gratification, and reward for effort were lived, not just learned as a concept. The income generated by our cattle was kept aside until we were adults and facilitated opportunities for us that few were blessed with.

Having grown up in the country, boarding school was always going to be on the cards. Our closest high school was over an hour away over rough gravel roads, and wasn't a viable alternative. My brothers and I had such different perspectives on boarding school; for me, it was always another adventure I looked forward to. As much as I loved the land, I wanted to experience so much more of the world and craved time around others. Both my brothers have wanted to be graziers their whole lives, so leaving home was a form of torture to them. Both are incredibly intelligent men but learning from a book never suited them, so school was never their happy place.

My desire for adventure extended well beyond only going away to boarding school. Rather than do a traditional "gap year" after school, I took part in a student exchange to Malaysia and spent the year of 1993 living with a Tamil family in Alor Setar. Picture a blonde-haired, blue-eyed, Caucasian girl from conservative rural Australia living in a developing city in an emerging Third World country, surrounded by mostly Muslim, Hindu, and Buddhist people. Those experiences opened my eyes to a much wider view of the world—one I am immensely grateful for!

My next adventure was a little closer to home—a university degree in Brisbane while trying to support my mother. After being unwell for many years, whilst I was in Malaysia Mum had been hospitalised with Chronic Fatigue Syndrome brought on by three simultaneous viral infections in her system. To begin with, I was mostly oblivious to how sick my mother was. In trying to integrate back into Australian life from Malaysia, my focus was on keeping myself on track. Because I had naturally looked so different when I was in Malaysia, simply walking down the street drew calls from the locals, as if I was a celebrity. Meanwhile, back in Australia, I was another normal human and the adjustment was pretty intense. I even had to open doors for myself again!

The Science degree I chose to do had a lot of flexibility and we were encouraged to have a clear direction in mind as we selected our subjects and designed our course of study. When you choose three different directions in three years, like I did, there's a lot of fun to be had but you end up with a degree that's not as immediately useful as it could have been. Looking back, it was absolutely perfect for the life I would live.

The years I spent in tertiary study were quite tumultuous. My mother was unwell for most of them, my parents separated in the middle of my second year, and their divorce was finalised by the time I graduated. When I started to look for work, my first thought was Perth or Tasmania. I figured moving to the other side of the country would give me enough space away from my family to unpack and decompress after all the craziness that had been my world. Instead, I landed a job with the Santa Fe Ski Area in New Mexico and went to the other side of the world rather than the other side of the country.

Another massive adventure began and I had so much fun! Working in childcare, I spent most days off snowboarding. By the end of the season, I could comfortably navigate the light powdery snow found only in the tree runs through the spruce forest. Santa Fe was another fascinating place to live and work. Margaritas and fajitas were standard fare and breakfast burritos were eaten most mornings.

At the end of the season, I used the income from some of my cattle to fund a six-month journey of self-discovery. I travelled nineteen thousand miles around Mexico, America, and Canada in a 1974 VW Kombi Camper I named Betty. Living frugally, I ate enough tuna on crackers to last three lifetimes, visited nineteen states within the United States, and crossed Canada from Niagara Falls to Victoria Island. When I arrived home, I discovered I owed money to my mother, who had been caring for my finances while I was away. So my next adventure was living with her and her new partner while I worked seven days a week to pay the debt off as soon as possible. That was interesting!

MY MESSY MIDDLE

Within just a few months of coming home from my trip through North America, I met the man who has now been my husband for over twenty-two years. Our journey together has had its fair share of challenges and successes. We have two amazing children and have weathered the storms of life that come with families, strong personalities, and some fairly extreme health conditions.

Our immediate family dynamic is quite traditional—not because we knew of nothing else, but because it enabled us to provide the life we wanted for our children. I had the honour of being a stay-at-home mother (SAHM) for about fifteen years, with the full support of my husband. We both wanted one of us to be present and available for our children when they needed us and chose to prioritise this over me chasing a career, or building a significant business, while they were young.

Being a SAHM was much harder than I expected but the choice to invest time and energy in our children at home, and choosing to parent in the way we have, is one I would make again in a heartbeat. It has not been perfect but I believe it's the best we could do for our kids. Each family has their own journey and needs to make decisions to fit with their personal life design, but the choice to sacrifice family holidays and fancy cars for the sake of having time with our children was the right one for our family.

We still had our fair share of challenges along the path. Taking physical care of the children was not so hard but the isolation and repetitive nature of the work was really difficult to resign myself to. I looked for more stimulation than only household duties, so became heavily involved in school and community activities, often had an entry-level, part-time job, and always ran at least one micro-business on the side.

These choices I made as a stay-at-home parent later led me to a crossroads in my journey, which is where I now shine as a coach for small business owners. In the process of dedicating so much of my world to being the support for our children, I forgot part of myself and lost sight of what else I wanted from life.

Imagine being in the messy middle of raising children, all your dreams packed up, shoved into a box, pushed under the bed, and stored for later. When the kids get older and need you a little less, the time comes to reopen that box. But, not only can you not get the lid open, sometimes it's impossible to even find the box! That's when you know that you've fallen into the trap of creating a life by default rather than by design. Perhaps out of necessity, perhaps because you didn't give much thought to it, the unconscious choices applied to all those little decisions in your life end up accumulating to create big results that you ultimately don't want.

CHOOSING WHAT TO CHANGE

Here presents a wonderful opportunity to start again. Firstly, it's important to review the past, then assess the present, before designing the future of your dreams. Once you know what your future and your Dream Life look like, next it's time to create your strategy, refine your systems, and build your dream.

Sounds simple, doesn't it? And in reality, it is. Not easy, but definitely simple. Allowing yourself the time, space, and grace to define your future is something few people will allow themselves. They're "too busy" to stop and take stock. It's easier to keep living a life on default, to keep accepting mediocrity. In doing so, they deny themselves opportunities to create more joy, fulfillment, and satisfaction in their world.

When I came to this crossroads in my own life, the Universe definitely conspired to point me in the direction of my dreams. Our eldest was in high school, the youngest in upper primary, and with their added independence, I had started looking for higher-level work opportunities. The frustration that came from working for others was extreme, so I kept exploring options.

Business coaching kept appearing in my periphery but I allowed my lack of confidence to stop me from pursuing the idea immediately. Then, following a training event in 2018, I caught up with Cassie, a friend I had known for many years. We chatted for hours over coffee about all things family, life, and business.

Cassie owned a hairdressing salon. When her children were small, she ran her business from home, and had expanded to commercial premises when the youngest started school. The change had created so many opportunities for growth and, at the time we talked, Cassie was facing some big challenges. She was stuck and stagnant in her business, held back by the systems she had in place. Her frustration was so great she had resigned herself to staying as a solo operator, expecting to cut hair alone until she fell one day with her scissors in her hands.

Her business model was in complete opposition to the life Cassie wanted to be able to lead. She was tied to her business five-to-six days a week, which left her no time to enjoy the money she was generating. At the end of our conversation that day, Cassie turned to me and said, "Terri, I've gotten more from you in the last three hours than I have from my business coach in the last three months. Will you be my business coach?" My mind spun into overdrive, the little voice on my shoulder that had kept me pinned for so long started shouting at me, and yet I heard myself say, "Sure."

At that moment my business, *Ten Thousand Dreams*, was born.

BRINGING DREAMS INTO REALITY

Cassie and I started coaching together soon after, unpacking all the parts of her business she was not excited about so we could find and implement new and better alternatives. As a way to help Cassie, and in response to patterns I noticed in others, I created a workshop system designed to give people the room to think, dream, journal, plan, and grow. The goal is to help people move from a state of fogginess to being crystal clear about the life they want to live and the business they want to create to facilitate this. Pulling together the most useful tools I had discovered in my thirty-plus years spent in active self-discovery, including content I had learned in my degree all those years ago, the work culminates in the creation of a Dream Board—a physical representation of the life you have designed.

When living the life you have designed, you're able to move forward with more certainty, confidence, and clarity. Ultimately this enables you to build your business to create the profit, impact, and fulfillment you're looking for balanced with the lifestyle you deserve.

This workshop has become the starting point for my clients when they begin coaching with me. Their Dream Board gives them, myself, and others a clear picture of where they are headed, so they can be better supported throughout their journey. A prominently displayed Dream Board gives your ideas space to germinate and sprout, so your dreams can grow into a form where you can live them. The beauty of this process is that it's easily repeatable. As you bring your current dreams into reality, it is simple to repeat the process and create a whole new set of dreams with a brand new Dream Board for the next phase of your life.

Prior to attending the workshop, I ask participants to take the time to step backwards, review their world, and journal all the ideas and memories related to every dream they ever wanted to accomplish. I invite you to do the same.

As you review your dreams, you'll find they will fall into one of four categories:

- Already achieved: these get a big tick alongside them

- No longer relevant: these dreams were once important to you but have been set aside as you've grown, matured, and become more aware of what you truly want

- Currently working on: these are the basis of your current goals

- Still important but you haven't started on these yet: these dreams have felt too big and overwhelming to start on, or will be relevant to you in another stage of your life

Once your vision is clear and your Dream Board has been created, it helps to underpin an additional level of confidence, enabling you to define and reinforce healthier boundaries, and gives you a clear direction so you can create the results you're looking for.

Take Cassie, for example. Once she set a clear direction around her life and her personal definition of success, we worked together to create smart strategies and establish structured systems for her business and home life. This clarity helped Cassie develop a stronger belief in herself and her capabilities, and made it easier to create and reinforce healthier boundaries in all areas of her life.

Cassie has transformed her world. She now has a team working in her business, has moved to a new, bigger premises, and created a space that is both welcoming and Instagram-worthy. She has outsourced services she dislikes and comfortably reduced her working days from six to four. Now living the life she only dreamt of when we started working together, Cassie has moved on to work with other coaches who are more salon-specific, and I am so incredibly proud of the changes she has made that we started together. It makes my heart smile to see clients like Cassie change their lives following these workshops and the coaching we do together. I know I'm making a difference in the lives of these people.

Every person I've ever worked with has a different definition of what their dream life looks like. Too many of us are living a life where we chase the standardised version of success and accept the mediocrity of a life lived by default. My mission is to help people to create and live their life by design.

And so I ask you to stop and think: What is it that you dream of? Are you living the life you have designed?

ABOUT THE AUTHOR

TERRI ADAMS-MUNN

Terri Adams-Munn started Ten Thousand Dreams after realising ideas and conversations she was sharing with business contacts were helping them transform their operations and achieve their goals.

Having grown up in Queensland on her family's cattle property, Terri was surrounded by people who lived their dreams every day. Unlike them, she didn't know what she wanted to do "when she grew up."

At forty-two, Terri finally worked out why she was put on this earth! Her mission is to help others discover their dreams and create the life and impact they were born for.

Terri's work is focused on small business owners who have become stuck and stagnant in their business, helping them to create clarity around the life they truly want to lead. She supports them through the process of transforming their personal boundaries and professional results so their dreams can become a reality.

CONNECT WITH TERRI HERE:

Website: www.tenthousanddreams.com.au

Free Gift: Seven Steps to Move You from Stuck and Stagnant to Motivated and Motoring www.tenthousanddreams.com.au/7Steps

For all socials and links: https://linktr.ee/TenThousandDreams

CLARA DEANS

BAPTISED TEN MONTHS BEFORE I WAS BORN

THE POWER OF RESILIENCE WHEN FACED WITH LESSONS IN LIFE

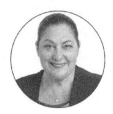

$\mathcal{T}$he first hint that possible trouble lay ahead occurred when I found out I was baptised ten months before I was born. At the age of twenty-seven, I had achieved three of four goals. The first was to have financial security; as a teacher I was making a good living. The second was to have a holiday house on the beach. The house I built was on an inlet, in a beautiful south-west coastal town in Western Australia. The third was to own a reliable car. I did. The fourth was to meet a man and marry by the time I was twenty-nine.

Life seemed to be going exactly as I planned until a cataclysmic event forced my life to change. I found myself questioning love and who I was, and learned that the only person I could truly rely on was myself.

It was in Australia in 1987 when I met an Irish man who I believed was the love of my life. He had one blue eye and one green, which I found mesmerising. One day, in a cute Irish accent, he asked me to marry him. Besotted, I said, "Yes."

Putting my entire heart and soul into a relationship, I sacrificed everything. We planned our future, preparing to live between Australia and Ireland on a two-year cycle. As professionals making a good wage, money wasn't going to be an issue.

Arranging a wedding on the other side of the world was no mean feat. But I was in the throes of euphoria, madly in love and ready to sell off everything and ride into the sunset with the man I loved. Family and friends' warnings were ignored. Emotions ruled me, not my head. The wedding was to be held in a beautiful church, chosen because of its spectacular floor to ceiling leadlight windows. They reminded me of the sails of the Sydney Opera House.

Five months prior to leaving for Ireland, a parcel arrived from the church. When opened, it revealed the signed, collated paperwork we had carefully prepared in order to get married in a Catholic church. Attached, was a simple message:

SORRY CAN'T MARRY YOU.

"Clara, do you realise you were baptised 10 months before you were born?"

Father Des O'Brien

Gobsmacked, I looked at the baptism certificate to read January, 1959. Then I looked at the birth certificate which said December, 1960— definitely a problem! It would have been laughable if it wasn't so serious! I couldn't believe my eyes. The birth certificate was wrong! I was born in November, 1959 but this document said otherwise.

I had to dig deep and demonstrate resilience to find a way. To find out more required contacting my estranged father, which meant navigating the anger and betrayal I felt towards him as a result of my childhood trauma. With some trepidation, I called him and asked the difficult questions. In a heavy accent, using self-taught English, he explained that he registered my birth on the same day as my sister, who was born three years after me. Speaking in broken Italian, they possibly did not understand him. He confirmed that I was indeed born in November, 1959.

On providing proof to *Births, Deaths and Marriages*, I obtained a birth extract and mailed the paperwork to the Irish priest via Express Post. Problem resolved. My fiancé and siblings all found it highly amusing. Little did I know that the date of my birth was to become an issue that would haunt me throughout my life. But that is another story.

Preparations for the wedding were in full swing. My wedding dress and bridesmaids' dresses were pre-made. Silk flower posies, bouquet, shoes, and undergarments were all beautifully presented in a very large white carry box. In all this, I gave little thought to the vision and goals I'd set for myself. Instead, I followed my heart and sold my car and holiday house to fund our new adventure. Something I would always regret. In allowing my fiancé to take control of everything, I unconsciously gave another person my power and lost myself.

Except when I chose the large white box containing all the wedding paraphernalia as carry-on luggage before boarding the plane. Asked to choose between them, of course I went for the box! On the airport floor I repacked. My priority was to protect the items in that box at all costs. After all, wouldn't you if you were the bride-to-be?

In hindsight, I probably should've been more practical but I didn't care. The white box I carried was treated like royalty. It was cumbersome and heavy. Strangers asked about it. And I revelled in the attention.

It was 2°C when we touched down in Copenhagen. We arrived, but our luggage didn't. Dressed in t-shirts and shorts, we headed out of the airport to a taxi that delivered us to our hotel. We both acknowledged a slight resentment towards the white box. I'd repacked the two windcheaters that would have been handy. Thank God for the heating in the taxi and the hotel.

What next you ask?

No one met us at Dublin airport. A phone call to his family created panic. They thought we were arriving the next day. His mother was renovating and the house was a mess. Apparently, our luggage had arrived at the hotel in Copenhagen but the concierge hadn't let us know.

Eight adults living in a two-bedroom, one-bathroom, mid-terraced, single-storey house meant sharing beds. Father and son. Mother and pregnant daughter. His younger sister and me. We barely spoke and the atmosphere was frosty! His father was the only one who was openly kind to me, but he worked all-day

Nothing went smoothly. From cars, to finding accommodation for visiting guests and family. The wedding day came but so did his sister's baby. The car broke down and the family pet passed away. Throughout it all, I was accommodating and allowed things to happen around me while I waited for the world to right itself.

Our honeymoon was a six-day sightseeing trip around Ireland before my husband went to London for work. Every week, he left on Monday morning and returned on Friday evening. At the beginning, this arrangement worked well. But being so far from home, friends, and family, I relied heavily on my husband to be my protector and ally. I believed that marriage was a partnership and I was doing it for us.

Within a few weeks, it became apparent that his mother wasn't happy. Her demeanour changed from sweet as pie if people were around, to mean and petty if we were alone. She informed me that he should have married an Irish girl, his ex-girlfriend to be precise. She insisted that I pay for my room and board, and expected me to do chores and assist with the baby for my keep.

Long walks and writing in my journal gave me solace during lonely days. I'd walk the streets looking for new places to explore. Leaving early in the morning and returning at dusk, I was deceitful in saying I had a job. My husband was angry as he expected me to keep his mother company but this practice of walking and journaling is something that I continue to do to this day. It became a part of my daily ritual.

I was relieved to join my husband in England. I regained a sense of independence and financial control; I was very glad to be working again. I also gained the realisation that being self-sufficient was essential to my happiness and wellbeing. Having autonomy to make decisions by regaining control of my finances was important for my self-esteem.

During the week we worked. On the weekend, we toured the countryside. But the fun stopped when his father was diagnosed with cancer. People-pleaser that I was, I became his carer on weekends in Dublin.

I was ecstatic when we bought a camper van because it meant we were finally beginning our European trip, travelling around France and into Italy via Genoa, where we stopped to get some cash.

On returning to our van, we found we'd been robbed. Thankfully, we'd kept our passports and licenses on us but the cash was gone. We agreed to use my credit card to fund the rest of our trip. Avoiding tolls, we drove all the way to the heel of Italy to visit my relatives who helped us to replenish items we'd lost. Finally, we had a chance to breathe!

Then we received bad news from Ireland regarding his father's condition and, with less than a month before the date of our return flight, we drove non-stop, each alternating driving and sleeping. Restrictions on our return flight tickets meant we had to return to Australia within a year of our departure.

Back in Australia a month later, we set up our house close to my sister and brother. Our focus was on him returning to Ireland so he could be with his dad and the family. Alone, he left for Ireland in April; it was seven months before I saw my husband again.

On his return, I booked a romantic getaway to Rottnest Island off the coast of Perth. Within two nights, he informed me he didn't think he wanted to stay married. It totally sideswiped me! I took off into the darkness to sit and cry! Later, with my bags packed, I headed to the dock. The next ferry to the mainland, twelve miles away, wasn't until morning. This is where he came to find me. He said he didn't mean it, that it had come out all wrong. It had been a difficult year for us both. He wanted us to take it slow, get to know each other again. He promised to do anything to make our marriage work.

He worked his Irish charm and convinced me to stay with him. In January 1991, when we celebrated our second wedding anniversary, I felt secure in my marriage. How gullible could I have been? Two months later it was over.

A message left on the answering machine. Our phone was about to be disconnected because the bill was over two thousand dollars and hadn't been paid for four months. I arranged to get a faxed copy. Our names were in the address bar, but the address wasn't our house. Instead, it showed a post office box in a different suburb.

A sense of dread invaded me. You know the feeling you get when you know that something is never going to be the same again? A repeatedly dialled number on the bill wasn't familiar so when I got home, I called it. An unfamiliar female voice answered and I slammed the phone down.

Robot-like, I headed for the post office, desperately needing to get there before it closed. As the "wife," I pretended I'd forgotten my key and was handed the mail over the counter. It was all for him. I could see bills, letters from Ireland, and bank statements. Accounts I had no idea existed. I opened one to find money—a lot of money was being deposited then withdrawn. Alarm bells were going off in my head! I was scraping pennies together while he was moving thousands through our joint account onto another.

I opened a letter from Ireland. It was from "her." The totality of his betrayal cut deep as I realised that during the last four months, he'd been living a lie. Fooling me into believing and trusting him. Meanwhile, his actions were that of a deceitful cheat and con artist. I'm not sure how long I sat there. The raw pain kept me silent as the tears silently fell. Then, somehow, I found strength to start the car and drive home.

I wanted to vent my anger! Enraged, I'd forgotten he was not there because he'd gone away to run a marathon that weekend. It would be two nights and a day before I could vent.

So I sprang into action fuelled by the spite and anger forged in my brain by the unpaid bills and her letter. Moving methodically from room to room, I went through everything in the house. Between swearing, cursing, and crying, I emptied, sorted, smashed, and stacked ready for boxing.

At daylight, I found the packing boxes I'd stored in the shed. My activity during the night had doused the rage, enabling me to make decisions. I was spent. The paperwork I'd uncovered had revealed other unpaid bills—rent, water, electricity. Over fifteen thousand dollars, including the credit card used in Europe.

Drawing on my resilience, calmly, methodically, and with precision, I began to box it all up. I moved his belongings onto the front porch but prepared my belongings and the rest of the house for removalists. I called an after-hours locksmith to change the locks, then headed around the corner to my brother's house.

One look at me and he called my sister. They let me cry and fall into exhausted sleep. When I woke, they helped me plan my next moves. *So blessed to have a supportive family.* On his return, my husband would find his possessions and the letter I wrote; I would not be seeing him again.

The financial shenanigans continued and left me destitute with a fifteen thousand dollar debt on my credit card. No place to live, no car. My one saving grace was that I had a teaching position. On the outside, I continued to function. Inside, grief and loss engulfed me.

I couldn't eat or sleep. I cried into my pillow at night. Obsessed, reliving everything over and over. Kicking myself for being so naïve. Ruminating on the events and asking "Why me?" and "What if?"

Mentally, emotionally, and physically a wreck, I wanted to get back what I'd lost. I wanted to erase the three years that had gone before. I'd been putting on a brave face but small cracks began to appear. They culminated with me having to attend mediation at work and being told to take personal leave to get help to manage my anger.

My family, also worried, told me I needed to seek help. It wasn't easy acknowledging I was in crisis again. I knew what I was going through because I had been paralysed by a major depressive disorder in my early twenties.

Feelings of hopelessness, fatigue, and low energy led to a diagnosis of "Adjustment Disorder with Depressed Mood," also called "Situational Depression" which means it isn't permanent. Typically, onset is within three months of the upset or trauma (in my case separation and divorce). The symptoms usually begin to recede within six months—if you get help.

Why am I sharing this? There is no shame in being depressed. *One in five women, and one in eight men will experience Major Depressive Disorder at some point in their lives.* (Australian Bureau of Statistics)

Going back into therapy was life-changing. It was my journey back into personal development and self-coaching. Showing resilience, I embraced uncertainty and engaged creatively with the unknown. It reignited my love of learning and reading. To take control of my life. To have a vision, set goals, and make plans to take action to achieve all dimensions of personal, financial and mental wellbeing. By being open and accepting of what came my way, I was saying yes to life—to the good, but also to the unpleasant. It filled me with courage, prompting me to experience each day feeling inspired and thankful for the simple things.

I used gratitude to assist me to focus on strengths rather than weaknesses. I learnt to welcome adversity. Discovering I was both resourceful and an expert on overcoming problems, I overcame challenges of a poor credit score and no access to a bank account or credit card.

Investing in myself, I took courses, workshops, and group therapy where I continued to build on my coping skills through connection. I cultivated strong relationships with other people who, in turn, nurtured hope and courage within me and helped boost my physical, emotional, and mental health.

I learned the tools, skills, and strategies to process and use so that I could strengthen my resilience and develop a personal philosophy that helped to support me. This gave me the determination to take actions that helped, not hindered, me. I became a lifelong learner, curious and open to new experiences.

Financially strapped and desperate, yet knowing it was the only way to avoid the poverty trap, I found creatively legal ways to make extra money. Budgeting, trying to make my personal ends meet on a limited wage, and working multiple part-time jobs to survive and avoid falling deeper into debt.

I took comfort in journalling my experiences and learning from them. I was authentic, spoke my truth, and managed my inner critic. Using self-reflection, recognising the disruption in my life, and taking time to think about how I needed to respond, I opted for solutions that represented my values and protected my interests. I permitted myself to challenge what and how I felt, and why. To learn to change. To grow and accept all of me. To embrace my failures and celebrate my wins. I discovered that putting myself first was not selfish. It was healthy.

Getting help, sharing my story, and writing everything down in my journal facilitated my recovery. To be resilient I had to take back the power from the person who had hurt me. I had to show forgiveness. It freed up my brain to focus on the things that made my life meaningful and brought me joy.

I am now able to help women who are living from day to day, job to job—and pay to pay! That's why I'm sharing my story.

Through my business, *The Welcome Philosophy*, I share my stories and the skills, tools, and strategies I learnt from these experiences to help women unlock the "fear and shame" that stops them.

As a wisdom activator and educator, I use the fear inside me as my motivation! I share that resilience starts with finding self-composure. Being in control by taking a few deep breaths and stemming the adrenaline surge. I am here to support women to recognise and build on their resilience.

By sharing insights about how I used resilience, my aim is to inspire women to take actionable steps for wellbeing every day of their lives. To stay optimistic and resilient, as I did, by:

- Remaining hopeful
- Remembering happy moments
- Having a supportive network
- Knowing their strengths.
- Having a purpose

- Believing in themselves

I run half-day workshops where I share the steps of *The Welcome Approach Model* to empower women to overcome their fear and shame and move forward, just as I did.

Putting yourself first is healthy—remember the oxygen mask on the aeroplane? It is why I teach women to take action and put themselves first. Their wants and needs matter. They don't need to change just to please others.

The first skill is to "love learning" and share what you learn. This is my passion. Why I model and teach rituals I incorporate into my daily life to maintain and achieve overall wellbeing and life balance.

Here's what I share:

1. I know what it is to be a woman who works hard, navigating each day the best way I can in order to provide the basics, the necessities of life, for myself and to ease the burden on my family.

2. What I used to overcome the "learned helplessness" of financial shame. That I too had stress and anxiety, head lowered in shame, occupied with the "day-to-day" pursuit of the mighty dollar. It lets them know they are not alone.

3. I used to live every day with joy and abundance and had *big dreams* of a wonderful future that I had designed. By investing in myself, I now make better goals so that different dreams happen.

Journalling is one practice I incorporate throughout all the interconnected dimensions of wellbeing: physical, emotional, financial, intellectual, social, spiritual, cultural, occupational, creative, and environmental. Another is the practice of walking (it saved me in Ireland) and I now offer my clients the opportunity to participate in a "Walk and Talk Meditation" in nature. We walk and talk, stop to breathe, get grounded, and remember to be grateful. Deeply listening, relating and storytelling, sharing understandings of what it feels like to walk through every day, living with stress and anxiety, head lowered in shame, occupied with the "day-to-day" pursuit of the mighty dollar.

A friend said, "Two ears are the most powerful organs of healing," and I agree.

Being patient and giving others my full attention when they're speaking, delaying judgment, and letting them complete their thoughts uninterrupted makes me a better listener—and therefore more resilient. It also helps them know they are not alone.

I can't reclaim my lost time. But what I can do is make sure that I don't lose the next twenty years without doing what I was born to do.

As for the saga of my birth certificate! It was an ongoing issue and has continued to haunt me throughout my life. It resurfaced to derail my ideal world. If you want to know more of that story you will need to join me in a workshop!

ABOUT THE AUTHOR

CLARA DEANS

Clara Deans is an experienced Speaker, Wisdom Activator, Educator, Mentor, and Storyteller. Through the power of story, her purpose is to support women to find the strengths within themselves to overcome any obstacles they are dealing with. She is the expert at overcoming everyday problems including financial woes, limiting beliefs, and feeling stuck.

Being in care (orphanage) for five years from the age of six was a positive experience that she attributes as being significant in supporting her to become the resilient person she is today. The Sister who was her major carer, gave her the foundation for living life to the fullest. She was given opportunities to pursue things that she found enjoyable, such as ballet and performing on stage, which cemented in her a love of learning new things. She loves to nurture this in others through her workshops and mentoring.

Clara offers walk-and-talk meditation along the beach, and 1:1 mentoring and group workshops. She is based in Scarborough, Western Australia where she lives with her husband and son.

CONNECT WITH CLARA HERE:

Free Gift: Ten journal prompts to enhance your wellbeing

For all socials and link to gift: https://linktr.ee/clara_deans

LENIN VONG

THE MAGIC OF SELF-BELIEF AND FORTITUDE

A BATTAMBANG GIRL'S STORY

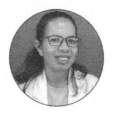

"The journey of a thousand miles begins with one step" -Lao Tzu

I love reading, especially Khmer fiction (Cambodian fairy tales).

I started reading those stories in 1990 when I was in Grade Five. At this point in time, my country was just ten years recovered from thirty years of civil war and it was still a baby step towards proper/formal education infrastructure. It was not easy for me to get access to books to read. The library had mainly a collection of old outdated books, the conditions on borrowing were quite strict, and opening hours were very limited. There weren't many bookshops and I had never been taken to one.

Born in a family of six children in a rural village in Cambodia, my father was a local government worker while my mother baked and sold traditional Khmer cakes. My father's work was around seven kilometers away from home, but due to poor road conditions and lack of transportation, he was only home once a month or even less. This meant mum played a role as both father and mother to look after all six of us.

My mum set very clear roles and responsibilities for each of us after school; my two brothers fetched the water from the pond, cut the wood, and harvested, and my older sisters cooked family meals, did dishes and other chores. I, as the fourth child, shared the household chores with my older sister and looked after my two younger sisters (one was five and one was one-year-old). My mum was busy making the Khmer cakes to generate a small daily income to feed the family. We did not have a clock back then, but we knew we must finish our tasks before dinner and after that, it was time to review our lessons from school and complete any homework. Daily study after dinner was compulsory for us and it came with my mother's daily motivational speech,

"You guys have the opportunity to study. Grab it. Your aunt and I did not have it because our parents could not afford education for all of us. We had to drop school to find the money for supporting the family's income and keeping your uncles in school. We women weren't encouraged to get education because eventually we would become a housewife and wouldn't work; so education is for men as they are the breadwinner of the family. I will do differently. I will try my best to keep all of you in school until you at least finish Year Twelve no matter whether you are my sons or my daughters. You were born to have equal education. And if you can go farther than Year Twelve, I will be even happier."

I felt very sorry for my mum but, to be honest, I also became bored with her daily repetitive speech. I doubted if we could achieve my mum's dream. She had only four siblings; two had to drop school. What about us? We were six and my family's income was no better, probably worse, than the income of my mum's family. At that time, physical punishment from parents was legal and acceptable in my country. So I studied because I was afraid of being blamed or punished by my mother. Luckily, we never failed our yearly exam. Even though we did not have individual comfortable bedrooms and were without electricity, (we shared light from an oil lamp to study at night) this achievement made my family highly recognized by the villagers; we were clever and hard-working kids.

In 1991, my older brother and sister finished Year Eight and had to go to high school in a town approximately ten kilometers away from home. My mum sent them to stay with my aunt and uncle to continue studying, so I inherited all their tasks and chores. We had to divide the same amount of household income into three portions, the first portion for household, the second for my brother, and the third for my sister. My mum felt stressed every day because of this new challenge. Sometimes, she threw her stressful emotions at my sister and me by cursing us with unpleasant words. Only reading story books could help me cope with this and entertain my life at those moments. Reading had become my hobby by then. I read all kinds of books, novels, tales, history, whatever that was available, because they helped me so much with all the situations that occurred.

"Done is better than perfect" -Sheryl Sandberg

In 1993, my family moved to live in the town when I was selected to join a class for outstanding students specializing in Khmer literature. Unfortunately, I had an accident, broke my ankle and had to skip class for three months to heal. With the help of traditional medicine from my uncle, I could go back to school after three months but, at first, I refused to go back and insisted on skipping class for the whole year. However, my mum assured me that it was fine to fail my yearly exam, but I had to go back to school and sit the exam at all costs. I had no choice but to go back, even though it felt hopeless. Nevertheless, I studied hard to catch up with what I had missed and to treat this exam as my own mock-up test. Can you imagine? Only three out of twenty-five students passed the exam and I was one of those three! Ten kids from my village sat at this exam and everyone failed except me. This result made me famous! After this fantastic accomplishment, I started my first English language lesson with a Buddhist monk together with other kids in the village. And so, my journey of learning a second language began.

"The best way to predict the future is to create it" -Abraham Lincoln and Peter Drucker

I entered working life in 2000 and, due to financial reasons, jumped between public and non-profit organisation sector jobs as a health worker. I also took breaks for further education.

After spending three years studying Nursing, I passed the state examination to work for the Government as a health worker at a health centre about fifty kilometers from home. That's exciting, hey? According to the government policy, new staff only received their wage once a year, in arrears. I accepted the job because it was better than nothing.

In order to survive while working without a salary for twelve months, I helped my colleague, a senior midwife, induce abortions. This service was very common during that time and the fee for performing the service was quite good, enough for me to wait for my annual salary to come. Abortion was legal back then because, with low rates of contraception, abortion was the only choice for most women who did not want to continue unintended pregnancies. Besides this, I also provided outpatient services to clients at home, when needed. Such private services were very common in the community where I worked, but these sources of income were very irregular. Therefore, I decided to come back home to do another one-year midwifery course in 2003, hoping it would bring me better job prospects. It also gave me the opportunity to be back with my family.

After graduating as a midwife, I worked as a social worker in one local NGO (Non-Government Organisation) to promote mental health in rural communities. My role was to conduct assessments in the village to identify if mental health support was needed. Through this, I learned that the underlying mental health issues for women in my society were domestic violence and gender inequality.

After one year of enjoying my income from the NGO, the news of my father's retirement arrived. This meant we would lose one source of family income and we needed to find other income sources to fill the gap. So I found another job, with a higher salary, at an international NGO called *World Vision Cambodia*. This job required a lot more commitment as I needed to study a lot of policies and guidelines for both technical and financial management. Most of the documents were in English so, to gain better proficiency in English, I resumed my weekend English course. Although my English is not perfect, I passed the IELTS (International English Language Testing System) test with an overall score of 5.5 (out of 9), which led to a life-changing opportunity where I travelled overseas for the first time.

This role with the International NGO allowed me to see opportunities for growth. I started to dream bigger. I wanted a different and higher position. So I decided to pursue a bachelor's degree while working with the expectation of promotion. I was right. With the combination of my degree and work experience, I was offered a position as Project Manager within the same organization but based in Phnom Penh, the capital city of Cambodia. It was good timing because my two younger sisters were getting a scholarship to do their bachelor's degree there as well, so the three of us relocated to Phnom Penh.

Working in the capital city was both exciting and challenging for me as an introvert. As a Project Manager, I worked alongside people within my organisation and government staff. When I had nothing to share in those meetings, I always got so anxious and wanted to escape, but I could not as my role required me to be there. There were very few women at those meetings. Those who were there didn't say much—including me! What *was* said was generally ignored, especially feedback that came from women. When the same thing was said by a man, it was readily accepted. I noticed that men seemed to have broader knowledge and were more outspoken and braver than women. So, after doing some self-reflection on my work-performance and job satisfaction, I decided I needed to improve my overall competency, including technical aspects of program effectiveness, English competency, and more active participation in meetings.

I started to explore learning opportunities and, fortunately, my friend shared information about a scholarship to study for a master's degree in Thailand. I did the research and quietly applied for it. Surprisingly, I passed all the application processes and was offered the scholarship. Off I went to Thailand to study for a Master of Health Social Science.

The opportunity to study in Thailand not only gave me the chance to pursue my education, but also opened my eyes to see society from multiple perspectives. The course is designed for international students from various countries such as Laos, Vietnam, Myanmar, Kenya, Mongolia, Bangladesh, Nepal, and Cambodia. I shared a house with classmates from Laos and Myanmar, so we had the opportunity to learn and share our own culture through cooking and eating together, and talking about politics, society, economics, people, weather, and so on from our own countries. We shared the challenges we faced in making our way to study in Thailand,

and we never forgot to be grateful for the life-changing opportunity gifted to us by the *Rockefeller Foundation*. Without their financial support, we would never be able to afford to study in a foreign country. On my return from Thailand in 2011, I worked at *World Vision International* in Cambodia again for a few years before I felt I needed to expand my horizon again.

ROAD TO IELTS (ACADEMIC) 6.5

"A dream doesn't become reality through magic; it takes sweat, determination, and hard work." -Colin Powell

Those who speak English as a second language will understand the challenge of upgrading the IELTS academic test score from 5.5 to 6.0 or from 6.0 to 6.5. The pressure is doubled when the upgrading target is within a short deadline.

In June 2015, after almost one year of working on my scholarship application, I received an email from the Chevening Scholarship program confirming that I was awarded the full scholarship to study in the UK under *one* condition—to obtain an overall and each band IELTS score of 6.5. I had to meet this requirement by the end of July 2015 or the award would not be valid. Oh my god, my excitement overlapped with anxiety! *How could I achieve this target score within this timeframe?* I had already sat the exam three times, and I had only achieved 6.0.

I told myself, "I can do this." But I knew I needed to be better prepared. Due to the limited number of candidates in Cambodia, the IELTS committee only organised the test once or twice per month and, to get a spot, a candidate had to book at least a month before the test date. I managed to book into the test in early July 2015, but this meant I only had one chance to get the 6.5 overall score. I was not confident and wanted to give myself more opportunity, so I registered for another test in Thailand a month earlier. It was a huge investment and commitment. So I bought preparation course material online and I studied hard to prepare myself.

Unfortunately, I still got only 6.0 on the test I did in Thailand. Crying inside, I felt hopeless. But with less than ten days to review lessons and to prepare for the final test in Cambodia, I didn't have much time for sadness and disappointment. So I took five days off work, studied rigorously, and went running regularly to keep myself sane. On the test day, I told myself it was pointless to be depressed. I knew I had done my best and was proud of myself. *Guess what?* The test result came after two weeks. I did it! "Candidate LENIN VONG, Overall Score: 6.5 (Listening: 6.5, Writing: 6.5, Reading: 6.5, Speaking: 7.0)." I was over the moon; I was going to study in London. My family, especially my mum, cried with joy and pride.

I arrived in London in September 2015 to do a master's degree of International Public Health Nutrition. It was exciting during the first few weeks with the new environment, amazing transportation infrastructure, clean streets, and magnificent buildings. Then culture shock rocked in and I became completely overwhelmed with the climate, food, travel, and communications at school, especially after going through all the study materials of the first four modules in Semester One. Sometimes I envied my classmates who spoke, read, and understood English as easily as they ate chocolate, while I was very slow and had to read a paper many times in order to understand it. I made all the way to the final exam and, eventually, I passed all the courses. I rewarded myself with one month travelling in the United Kingdom and several countries in Europe and then closed off by running a twenty-one kilometre race before I returned home. I have practiced running regularly since then.

On 28 September 2016, I returned to Cambodia. On my way home, I received a message from a former colleague who asked if I was interested in applying for a job. But I decided to work as a freelancer for some time, and spent a two-month break with my family before I applied to be a consultant at a local NGO. They offered me the opportunity to lead a project to design a community-based nutrition program in the remote province of Kratie, in the north-eastern part of the country. The people of Kratie are poor and a lot of mothers and children are malnourished. I was so happy to return to work with *Community Health Workers* to design their project to rehabilitate malnourished children and prevent future malnutrition. Every day for a month, the local NGO worker took me to the village on his motorbike to work with women and children. Despite my joy in this job, my family—especially my mum and my brother—felt so disappointed. They said I should have been working in a big office in

Phnom Penh instead of that remote area. They kept calling to repeatedly express their sadness but this did not stop me and I finished this project successfully. Later on, the Director of this local NGO invited me to be the long-term Technical Advisor for their organization, and they continued to seek my advice when they faced challenges throughout the project implementation, as well as when designing a new project.

After doing several other short-term projects, I was offered a full-time consultancy position at *World Bank* where I was tasked to work with the team to pre-design a nutrition project for the country. This was the first big nutrition project in Cambodia and I was so proud to be part of this team for eighteen months.

After this project, I received an offer to be a full-time Technical Specialist at *Save the Children Cambodia*, where we worked on adolescent health and nutrition in schools. During this exciting opportunity, I worked directly with young adults to develop school and community campaigns to promote a healthy diet. I was so happy to see those young people work together to make their campaign as effective as they expected.

Not long after that, there was another exciting opportunity at the *World Health Organisation* (WHO) to work with the Ministry of Health and the Ministry of Education to promote health and nutrition through life cycle. I decided to leave the lovely *Save the Children* to join *WHO*, with the expectation that I would have influence on the policy changes for the whole country! My expectation was fully achieved because I had a chance to work with the School Health Department under the Ministry of Education to promote healthy snacks in primary school and advocate for the elimination of unhealthy drinks and snacks.

In late 2019, I decided to leave *WHO* to join *UNICEF* as a Health and Nutrition Officer. Here, I work with the Ministry of Health and other relevant Ministries to make sure that all Cambodian children under two-years-old receive vaccinations to prevent diseases. At first, I was so overwhelmed with the new area of expertise required in this new job. But then the Covid-19 pandemic in 2020 became an opportunity for me to be more resilient and I started to love this job every day, regardless of workload and challenging moments.

As I reflect on my journey this far, I am filled with pride at the perseverance that has been instilled in me by my mother. Education and perseverance lead you to your goals, regardless of where you come from. You can be who you want to be.

I now have a voice at the table, whereas in previous years I didn't. Having applied myself to develop my skills means that, through the work I do, I can now make a difference in the lives of many.

If I can leave you with anything to inspire hope in you, it is this: Nothing limits your education. If you dream about it, strive for it, and walk into it, you will make it. Step out of your comfort zone, and you will make a difference in your life, and to the people around you. I believe in you, now it is time for you to believe in yourself.

ABOUT THE AUTHOR

LENIN VONG

Lenin Vong is a skilled health professional with extensive experience in nursing, midwifery, and public health nutrition for over ten years.

After completing her nursing training, she began working for the Cambodian government in health facilities in remote rural areas, where she gained valuable experience in healthcare delivery and patient care.

Seeking to expand her skills and knowledge, Lenin pursued a Diploma in Midwifery, expanding her work to support women and children in disease prevention through behavior change promotion. Through this work, she gained a deep understanding of the healthcare needs of these populations and honed her ability to provide compassionate care in challenging situations.

To advance her career, Lenin completed a Master's Degree in Public Health Nutrition from Westminster University in the United Kingdom. Both her experience and education have spurred her further on her mission to improve public health outcomes, especially among vulnerable populations through her work with UNICEF.

CONNECT WITH LENIN HERE:

LinkedIn: https://kh.linkedin.com/in/lenin-vong-b35808174

For all socials and links: https://linktr.ee/battambang_girl

JACQUI PENNY

STAIRWAY TO HEAVEN

STEPS TO TRANSFORM DEBILITATING FEAR INTO PURPOSE-FILLED BLISSFUL FREEDOM

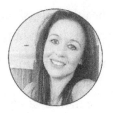

"A journey of a thousand miles begins with the first step." -Tao Te Ching

Coming down the stairs thirteen years ago, hemorrhaging internally, clarity hit me as I surrendered to something much bigger. I should have died that day but I'm here to talk about that walk down the stairs, that brink of death moment, because I believe the message I received was not for me alone. It was for you. Yes you! The amazingly precious soul reading this book, and in particular, this page, this very line. That first step on my stairway to heaven, both literally and figuratively, transformed my life. It guided my way, just as my purpose is to Make A Difference by guiding you. With my six easy-to-follow steps, it *can* be done. Transformation from suffering fear, endless anxiety, and people-pleasing paranoia will come. After that moment of clarity I received on the stairs of my Auckland home, I began my journey of truth towards freedom.

Unfortunately for me, however, it did feel like a thousand miles before I reached that point. To put it plainly, I had lived my whole life often in a state of paralyzing fear. I was plagued by anxiety before I knew to call it that, in a way that was extreme, to say the least.

Living in this world, the very one you now inhabit, was a daily struggle. No—that's not true—I could handle a daily struggle but my reality was an hourly struggle. At times I found it a seeming impossibility to get from one minute to the next. From as early as I can remember, I constantly worried and ruminated on catastrophes. *Why?* Because I let the world dictate how I felt about myself and internalized any perceived criticism to the point of internal anguish. *Do you do this?*

I did, however, know one thing. I did not fit into the world as I was experiencing it. As a result of this perception, by the age of ten my stress levels had already compounded to the point where they were affecting my young self in the most direct way—physically. Nothing would make me sit up and take notice more than the first and the last of these experiences. This is what led me to look back eventually at the repeating patterns I formed. Yes, the last time was that moment on the stairs—"Step One," I will get to that I assure you. But, because I want you to become as driven to effect change within yourself as I was, I need to take you back in time.

On a day that started out no differently from any other, I made a discovery that my innocent young soul remembers so vividly, it could have been made of translucent, shining, white light. Sometimes I think it was. They do say the darkest moments come before the dawn, and this has always proven true for me.

I encourage you to think of your own patterns as you read this. These are often like the threads of a finely-crafted tapestry interwoven throughout your life, allowing cracks to appear and light to flood in. Hence "Step Two"—learning to overcome these patterns—was developed.

BECOMING INVISIBLE

Everything that had ever been mirrored back to me from people who had casually put me down, bullied me, or made me feel small, was finally affecting my health. This took the form of losing my hair which, upon discovery, I immediately attempted to control via developing an eating disorder.

I began to call my increasing bald spot, "It." "It" was a silent parasite that fed on the stress I felt as a result of being "It's" host. This, in turn, only made my eating disorder grow in severity.

By the age of fourteen, I had lost any remaining shred of self-respect. "It" was never talked about at home (at least not directly to my face), within my family, or at school. Maybe it was the enduring shame "It" represented, but I closely guarded this secret, even though it was becoming less of a secret every week. At least two years passed before it was finally addressed, out loud by my mother, in the form of the humiliating exposure of 'It' during a visitation to my doctor to get a referral to an unbearably sterile specialist's office. I was not given any answers, only informed of the possibility that there was a 60% chance of 'It' happening again, even if my hair eventually did grow back.

At school, of course, there were many whispers and conversations hidden behind hands during that time; something said slightly loud enough to be overheard but never directly to me—which left me powerless to respond. Those early years I spent at an all-girls' high school were insufferable.

So, once again, I shrank and withdrew. I became small. I was being taught that being female meant I had to look a certain way and I did not look it, no matter how hard I played my "eat-nothing-for-days-on-end" game. Eventually, I was unable to hold out any longer and caved, leaving an ashamed shell.

My grades, which were formerly very good, dropped to the point where I gave up trying to even listen in the classroom. If I didn't try, then I wouldn't be disappointed. I basically spent my days listening to my internal criticism, often mirrored from those around me, or what I projected onto them. By this time, I was outwardly being bullied with notes telling me exactly how ugly I was being strategically slipped into my locker just in case I wasn't already aware I was such an oddball.

During the day, I often left school and went home. If my older brother came home from school at lunch time, or earlier than expected, I hid in my closet. On good days I stayed in the toilets, often crying quietly until school finished. My self-esteem plummeted to an all-time low until I eventually became what I had set out to become—invisible. The smaller I made myself, both figuratively and literally, the better.

I had become so small, quiet, and shy, that any interaction resulted in a reaction that varied from a flaming, red-cheeked blush to panic attacks, often while experiencing simultaneous, uncontrollable trembling.

But being ignored was the worst. I lost all sense of Self, a key element of mastering "Step Three." Before I learnt to fully embody this, I allowed the external world to dictate what I saw when I looked in the mirror. I didn't see beneath the exterior, and what I did see clearly didn't live up to the expectations living by the world's rules was having on me. In reality, I had placed these expectations on myself long before 'It' had taken residence. But I didn't see that then.

Being invisible and small felt as if I didn't exist at all. For three long drawn-out years I merely mechanically witnessed daily life. I felt ugly, I felt fat, I felt unworthy. I felt worse than unworthy—I felt worthless. Powerless.

In retrospect, it's interesting to see how this tapestry thread often habitually reared its head until I made permanent changes through my own perception. Something I was unaware I had control over the entire time; this is explored in "Step Four."

My hair did grow back, eventually. And it did not fall out again, despite the horrifyingly haunting statistic young-me was insurmountably faced with. And I did get over my eating disorder, eventually.

How? Every night when I prayed that I would not wake up in the morning, I was initially unrelenting in this request. Instead of the line, "If I die before I wake, I pray the Lord my soul to take," I said to my young, innocent, perfectly-whole Self, "Please may I die before I wake and please, oh please, take my soul."

When I think of my small Self saying this, I want to reach out to her, beyond the years, and give her a hug. The biggest hug I could possibly give any innocent child who does not know how very wrong she truly is, or the fact she is not alone. I often do this in my daily meditations, which are part of "Step Five." I yearn to let her know that, in time, she will learn this. That she will develop concrete tools to help others, such as yourself, who suffer from paralyzing fear, anxiety, and/or depression. That through the lessons she learned many years later as she internally bled into her abdomen, on a staircase, a seeming world away from the small child she was, that her little child had remained hidden all along. But for now, I feel that little child's pain so incredibly deeply, just as I feel yours.

MYSTERIES REMAIN

Part of me wonders if I could sense my older, wiser Self even back then. Because one day, I felt ever so slightly more guided, and gradually started to pray differently. I started to say, "if" I die before I wake. Other times, I would just be. In my prayer I felt safe, as though comforting arms were wrapped around me. Alternative thoughts came to mind. I began to see life from an ever so slightly altered perspective, different from the "reality" I had created, supposedly dictated by the world I inhabited, that hadn't actually changed at all. I realize now that I had accidentally begun to "meditate," even before I knew this word existed. I meditated on the fact that there might be hope. Perhaps I could choose to be different and take action? I entertained the tiniest possibility that I could choose to be whoever I wanted to be; although I wasn't fully *there* at this point, I was heading in the right direction.

The questions of, "Why did 'It' happen to me?" and, "Why do bad things always happen to me?" gradually changed. They became, "What can *I* do to physically change myself?" and, "What can *I* do so I don't feel so bad every single day?" Even though I continued to wake up disappointed that my prayer to die in my sleep had yet again not worked, at least it didn't feel quite as much like Groundhog Day.

Thus began the process of change. But it has been a long one over many years. I was, however, on a path forward, which felt good. And it did work for a time. I started to read books on good health and ate healthily instead of destructively. By the time I reached my sixteenth year I was exercising, listening in class, and resumed trying to do well. I became physically and mentally stronger. The self-criticism continued but at least my hair had grown back entirely.

I do not want you to endure the years of wrong turns I took. I want to make a difference so that the "quick fix" attempts to change myself, to please others, and to please the unfailingly critical voice of the ego, do not continue with you. This egoic voice often poked its spiny finger between my eyes when hurdles inevitably came my way. During these times I resorted to those old same patterns of trying to find a way to fix it from the outside in, rather than the inside out.

And once again, I would find myself shaking in my boots any time I was outside my comfort zone, which was generally when I was around people. Any people. Often, family was no exception as I created dialogues of what others *must* be thinking about me.

At first this was to prove my Chemistry teacher wrong when she said, flat out, that I would not pass my major exams, and that my parents and I should "just prepare for that." It helped that I became angry. Angry at her, angry at the girls at school who ignored me, just angry. So I decided to prove her wrong. To prove them all wrong. I was still living according to others' opinions of me, but I decided their opinion would change if I changed myself, and as this gradually happened, I did receive some positive feedback to fuel my embryonic Self-worth.

I felt some pride in myself. But this pride was based on achieving things by the world's standards. So, whenever I fell short of the expectations I had for myself, the paralyzing fear came back with abundance. I was so used to looking outside myself for external validation that I could not see what was there all along. I was always whole; I was always complete. Nothing else needed to be done. I was perfect the way I was.

If I had realized this then, all the subsequent years spent chasing vice after vice would have not happened. But I was stubborn. I had to learn the hard way what I knew deep down all along. I was a good person. But words often used to describe me, such as kind, caring, and compassionate, unfortunately didn't cut it. I wanted to be dynamic, outgoing, one of the confident loud girls who would shout their opinions for the whole world to hear.

Hence my life went in habitual, self-torturous cycles. Until at last, I used up all my external 'solutions' and was left, simply, with *me*. By the time I married in my late twenties, numerous quick fixes had dismally and tragically failed. My youngest child was three-years-old by the time stress began to attack my body for the final time, in the form of an H.pylori infection. This was not my first infection. My immune system was "surprisingly low for someone of my age," as was my poor circulation, high blood pressure, and general well-being. At least that's how the doctors saw it. They didn't get the connection with stress. Neither did I.

I developed ulcers from this bacterium attacking my stomach lining and agonizing pain resulted. Initially, I didn't listen to what my body was screaming to me at the top of its lungs. I didn't call an ambulance when I vaguely sensed the tearing sensation of my duodenum and stomach during the previous night, spilling into my abdomen cavity. I was too socially awkward to "put out" an ambulance crew. "The pain will subside," I told myself, "just ride it out." I thought this was simply another cycle. Only this time it wasn't. My lowered immunity, thanks to my debilitating anxiety, was almost certainly about to cause my death.

That prayer from all those years ago was finally being answered. I had manifested what my subconscious had wanted all along. That terrified little girl who still resided in me was, once again, presiding *over* me.

MY HEAVENLY STAIRS

It was a Monday morning when I awoke semi-conscious. I was close to death. But I had a life—three beautiful young children and a husband who loved me deeply. Thankfully, knowing I was not well, he had not yet left for work that day. My older two children were at school and kindergarten leaving just my three-year-old little girl playing happily downstairs.

I was barely functioning; only enough to experience the ceaseless waves of excruciating pain that crashed over and engulfed me. Once again, just as when I was that little girl, I prayed.

What happened next shouldn't have happened at all. I shouldn't have been able to stand. Shouldn't have been able to struggle to pull a skirt over my confusingly distended belly. I stood swaying in my bedroom, gazing down at my enormous stomach. I looked nine-months pregnant. How could that be? I hadn't eaten all weekend. I needed help.

Somehow, I stumbled out of my bedroom, made it across our hall, and began the seemingly insurmountable journey down the stairs. My gaze was drawn out the nearby window, to the sun streaming inside, when it dawned on me. I could not handle this anymore, this was bigger than me. I could not handle the pain, the nausea, and the debilitating anxiety and subsequent depression that had plagued my life. So, I did the only thing I knew how to do. I handed it over to a higher power. For me, that was God.

In those crucial moments when you need something other than yourself, everyone becomes a believer. For you, that higher power may be Mother Nature, the Universe, the intelligent driving force that regulates the world, or what I like to call "all those things combined"—your individual innate purpose for being. Surrender, what I call "Step One," was incredibly liberating.

It's not until you become totally unencumbered by fear that your purpose, your sense of power, is free to appear. Many cannot get past this hurdle. Others must suffer before we gain insight. I plan to guide you out of your pain. Where the cracks in your life occur, a light will shine through—if you are ready. If you have reached that point of no return, that point of surrender.

You have to choose. Are you going to get busy living? Or get busy dying?

On my heavenly stairs, I finally admitted this situation was bigger than me. Sweating profusely with a high fever, I was going into septic shock. Droplets ran down my forehead into my eyes, mingling with my tears. My core was on fire. I was not going to be able to act, talk, pretend, or alter my way out of this one; this was the big league. In that moment I knew without a shadow of a doubt that it was the day, if not the hour, the moment, that I would die. I experienced what can only be described as *knowing*.

It was about something powerful, and loving, and pure bliss. It was contained in the sunlight that streamed in the window. This happened in an instant, although time was no longer important. I knew that if I surrendered, I would be okay. Everything in my life would naturally, easily, and effortlessly change for the better. I would be free.

Now, I was close to death as confirmed by my doctors later. I shouldn't have been able to walk out of my bedroom internally hemorrhaging blood, burning rancid stomach acid, and bile into my increasingly distended abdomen cavity.

The knowledge I experienced in that instant has never left me. It was an amber-light-filled clarity like I'd never experienced, and I knew it to be true. It was real. I was not on drugs. The endorphins for my pain were long past trying to kick in, this was purely a spiritual awakening.

The minute I admitted defeat and asked for help I was overcome. I have had many glimpses since that day, often in meditation, or when I'm connecting with people by showing up authentically as me, not as a guarded equivalent. Or when music touches my soul like only music can.

Once we know something to be true, we never unknow it. I felt two shapes at my side who guided me down the stairs. My three-year-old daughter assumed we were playing "zoo animals" when she appeared just in time to see me reach the bottom of the stairs and crumple onto all fours. Somehow, I crawled across the hall on cool tiles, my daughter doing the same as she made roaring lion noises. As we made our way into our expansive kitchen, where my husband was making breakfast, I felt my life draining away. Yet I managed to breathe one word, "Ambulance."

Leaning against a nearby sofa I closed my eyes, blocking out the world.

At times, I came to and reassured the ambulance officers that I was going to be okay, telling them not to worry as I heard them inform the emergency registrar I was "Code 1" before passing out again. I even informed the Surgical Registrar in the Emergency Resuscitation room that I was going to be okay. I had knowledge that they did not. I had seen the way past this as clearly as if I had been watching a sparkling amber movie screen that pointed the way. Even when they brought my husband and confused toddler in to "say goodbye" before what was apparently considered a futile attempt at emergency surgery, I reassured them all.

It wasn't until I woke up in hospital that the gravity of my experience hit me. The ambulance crew took the rare step to visit me the following day, making an exception to see for themselves that I was still very much alive.

From that day onwards, I have managed my stress levels through surrendering myself daily, meditating, and entertaining a perspective on life that is 180 degrees from my previous "outside-in" view of the world. This perspective has now become second nature. As a result, I gained insight into my purpose for being uniquely me; the final step on my "stairway to heaven."

I got busy living. I want you to get busy living too. Believe me, you won't look back.

I created my six simple steps for people who remain stuck in fear, to provide a roadmap for getting out of that state to a place of freedom. A place where purpose lives and leads to bliss. Where fulfillment lives. Where love lives. *Why don't you join me here?*

Visit me at *www.healingplace.co.nz* for information on how to embody my simple "Six Steps to Gain Freedom from Fear." Experience the peace of a purpose-driven life. An existence you can only begin to imagine. *You can create it.*

ABOUT THE AUTHOR

JACQUI PENNY

Jacqueline is a Holistic Life Coach, Meditation Teacher, Creative Life Writer, and qualified professional Journalist. She empowers women to live their desired lives, believe in themselves, and take risks to pursue their dreams. Her coaching focuses on developing self-belief, courage, and inner peace.

With a BA in English and a postgraduate Master's degree in Creative Writing, Jacqueline has over twenty years of experience as a Journalist in feature writing, content writing for newspapers, magazines and business content. She is a US-certified holistic Life Coach, skilled in creative life writing, meditation, and holistic health and mental practices.

Jacqueline combines her passions to serve her clients, helping them fulfill their lives and raise the planet's vibration. Based in Auckland, New Zealand, she finds daily inspiration walking on the beach.

With her diverse expertise and genuine commitment to personal growth, Jacqueline brings a unique approach to coaching, writing, and teaching, uplifting individuals and fostering positive change.

CONNECT WITH JACQUELINE HERE:

Website: http://www.healingplace.co.nz

Free Gift: Self Awareness Checklist to kick-start your journey. http://www.jacquelinepennyauthor.com

LinkedIn: https://www.linkedin.com/in/jacqueline_penny_634861265/

DR. KATE LUND

RESILIENT PARENTING

HELPING KIDS THRIVE
WITHIN THEIR OWN UNIQUE CONTEXT

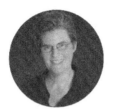

*T*he final race of the season's second rowing regatta was about to

begin. Sunlight glistened on the water as the boats lined up at the starting line. Among the rowers were my fifteen-year-old sons, Alex and John. Alex, who had started rowing last year, sat in the center of the A boat. This was John's first year, and I knew he was eager to catch up with Alex's skill level. Both had been practicing on the rowing machine every chance they got. At night, they fell asleep brainstorming strategies to improve their times.

Although they are twins, Alex and John are very different. Alex has always enjoyed learning about various topics at school and playing a wide range of sports. He commits himself and does well at just about everything he puts his mind to, both in the classroom and on the field.

Accomplishments don't come as easily for John; he struggles to block out distractions, manage his time, and keep himself motivated at school. Lately though, he's been exploring the unique context within which he is free to find and follow his own passions and make his talents shine. John entered his freshman year very unsure of the activities he wanted to try outside the classroom. He joined the cross-country team in the fall, but struggled to build stamina as a runner and feel connected to the team. While a bit discouraged, he forged ahead and joined wrestling the next season. Although exciting at first, it became clear as the bruises started to emerge that wrestling was not a good fit for John. Again, he was a bit discouraged, but he pushed on and decided to give winter crew conditioning a try.

Things clicked for him and he has not looked back. John's growing passion for crew is an example of how sticking through the hard moments has helped him realize his strengths in a new way. By pushing himself out of his comfort zone, taking risks, and trusting his physical abilities without worrying or comparing himself to others, he has recognized strengths he did not know existed. Each time he hits a goal or personal record (PR) on the rowing machine or during a lake run at practice, John is building belief in himself and his abilities in a new and exciting way. This is having a positive impact on him not only in crew, but in the classroom, and in social and family relationships.

John is learning that it is okay to take your time to find the path that feels right, and not just do things because others are doing them. He is learning that this is a much more satisfying way to get through life than trying to live by other people's external standards. What this means is that he's been finding his intrinsic motivation and figuring out ways to navigate the challenges he faces in his own creative ways. He's also been learning new tools and techniques to develop his skills and accomplish the goals he sets for himself. Most importantly, he is learning to believe in himself and all that he is capable of.

This kid has been making amazing progress. For example, he was placed in a math class that was a little beyond his skill level this year. It was hard to watch him struggle at first. I thought about meeting with his teachers and asking them to transfer him to a class that was more his speed. But since John didn't suggest it himself, I didn't bring it up.

Instead, I guided him to make realistic goals with his unique context in mind, and asked him to come up with concrete steps he could take to make sure he learned as much as he could while he was in the class, no matter what grade he might end up with on his report card. John decided to dedicate half an hour each afternoon to studying math. He also tried to study with a tutor, but that didn't work out. She was chatty, which turned out to be a little distracting, and then toward the end of the session she became impatient and did the work for John after breezing through explanations. At first, John blamed himself for not benefiting from the tutor's help, but I pointed out that there might be a more productive way for him to learn—meetings with the teacher, for example.

When he stopped working with the tutor, he found that he was able to focus better and retain more of what he was learning. He made a valuable discovery about himself: that taking the time to work things out on his own was a much better way for him to master the concepts than watching the tutor do his homework. He decided that his time was better spent at weekly after-school meetings with his teacher, where he asked questions about concepts and troubleshot areas where he was having difficulty.

On the day of the mid-term exam, John was ready for his ride to school a good five minutes early. He leaned against the armrest of the couch, his full backpack at his feet, and watched the street outside.

"Are you nervous about the test?" I asked.

John just grinned and shrugged. "Pretty sure I've got this," he said.

I was feeling pretty certain too. This was the hardest I'd ever seen him work on anything school related. He had stuck to the commitments he made, spending at least half an hour studying quietly at the kitchen table every day. He kept all of his meetings with the teacher, no matter what else came up. When the idea of hiring a tutor turned out to be less than fruitful, he was able to switch gears and pivot to another strategy instead of getting discouraged.

When John got home from school, he gave me his usual, "Hi, Mom," and went to the fridge, as if this were any other day.

"So... how did the test go?"

"It was hard," he said.

"Did you get to go into the testing room?"

"Yeah. But there was still a lot of noise. There were a lot of people in there. It was hard to focus." As he talked, he lined up a pack of bologna, a loaf of bread, sliced cheese, and mayo on the counter.

"Sounds nerve-wracking," I said.

"It was. I got pretty worried." I watched him carefully alternate the bologna and cheese on a slice of bread after spreading the mayonnaise.

"Did you slow down, the way we talked about? Did you take your time instead of rushing through it?"

"Yeah. I did that."

"Well, it sounds like you did your best, John."

He shrugged. "We'll find out how I did on Monday."

"We already know how you did!" I reminded him. "I'm really impressed with how hard you worked, and how you stuck with everything you said you would do. You did great!"

"Yeah, yeah," John waved my praise away with his finished sandwich and carried it out to the patio.

The following Monday, John came home and said, "You know that test?" He had his poker face on.

"The math test last week? Did you get the results?"

"I got a C-!" His brow was furrowed. "I didn't think I was going to ace it or anything, but..."

"Dude! That's awesome! So much better than the first test, which was an F, right?"

"Sure, but..."

"But what?"

"Aaron got a C and now he's *grounded*!"

"His context is different, right? You guys are not the same people."

"That's true," John agreed. Aaron was a friend of John's who had been in advanced math classes since fifth grade.

"Think about the progress you've made! Do you think you can keep this momentum going all the way until the final?"

John relaxed and smiled. "Sure!"

"Alright," I pulled out a chair for him to join me at the kitchen table. "Let's revisit your strategy. What were the things you did that helped the most for this test?"

"Well..." John rubbed his chin. "The meeting with my teacher really helped. And I did slow down and take my time on the test."

"So you're going to keep meeting with your teacher, right? And keep studying at the same time every day?"

He nodded.

We brainstormed a few other things he could do, like stopping by the math lab after school and arranging for a quieter environment to test in. By the end of the conversation, John was excited to go into the last half of the semester with a few proven strategies, a few fresh new ideas, and the challenge of a test score to beat.

I was proud of the maturity John demonstrated in setting his own goals, finding ways to keep motivated, and continuously improving his performance in math. Still, I worried that he might be hard on himself if he didn't beat his own expectations in the regatta that day. Rowing is a difficult sport that requires excellent strength, stamina, and team communication as well as coordination. Even Alex, who has a knack for making most things look easy, struggled with rowing during his first year.

I've always worked to instill in my kids a belief I hold dear—that winning or losing doesn't matter nearly as much as building strong relationships, developing skills, and having fun. Each child has their own range of abilities and possibilities—their own unique context in which to discover their zone of genius. When we stop comparing ourselves to others and learn to find joy in our own abilities, we are free to discover the talents and passions that are unique to each of us as individuals. This philosophy has been ingrained in me since my own childhood.

I grew up with a rare condition that caused problems with the circulation of my cerebrospinal fluid. The shunt that helped drain the fluid from my brain necessitated long hospital stays, a series of funny haircuts, a heavy hockey helmet that I had to wear when I played sports, and large, thick glasses. I grew up knowing that the context of what was possible for me was very different from that of other kids my age.

I remember the moment I realized I would never have a "normal" childhood, no matter how hard I tried to wish my condition away. I was at a birthday party in a neighbor's backyard. They had a trampoline, and all the other kids my age were jumping on it. I was standing off to the side, between the adults who were gathered around the barbeque and the smaller kids who were coloring with crayons at a folding table. As an eight-year-old, all I wanted was to tumble around with the other kids who were bouncing into the sky and shrieking with glee.

As soon as the adults went inside, I climbed onto the trampoline and jumped as high as I could. It was so much fun! Then everything started spinning. I vomited over the side of the trampoline, and continued to throw up for the next week.

Until that incident on the trampoline, my parents had a difficult job redirecting my attention away from the competitive sports and rough-and-tumble activities I longed to participate in. What made things easier was that they were also diligent about pointing out activities that were possible for me so that I wouldn't spend a lot of time dwelling on the things I couldn't do.

When things were going well, my parents treated me like the child I was instead of the condition I happened to have. They didn't shield me from the challenges of life. Instead, they made sure I had the tools I needed to overcome the obstacles I faced, and they encouraged me to look forward to the possibilities that opened up for me on the other side of those challenges. I was fortunate to benefit from their wisdom.

My dad noticed that I enjoyed throwing a tennis ball to the family dog, for example. When the dog got tired of playing fetch, I would bounce the ball against the wall of the garage and then run wildly to catch it. So he bought a pair of rackets, took me to the tennis court at our neighborhood park, and together we learned how to play tennis. I had a lot of fun developing my skills, setting goals for myself, and beating my records one by one. I played competitively with other kids too, and even captained my high school team and played in college.

I brought home a few trophies, although I rarely placed first in tournaments. But those types of victories were never the point. On the tennis court, I proved to myself over and over again that I could accomplish goals most people would have thought impossible. For me, that was thrilling!

Fast forward to the year I graduated from college when I rode my bike fifteen hundred miles from Seattle to Denver as part of a group called *Cyclists Ending Hunger*. This was something nobody who knew me as the downtrodden little girl in the big glasses and funny haircut would have thought possible.

That bike trip was arduous! I'll never forget pedaling into the headwinds across Idaho, dead last in the group. I was so far back, the second-slowest rider looked like a speck on the horizon. But I was happy! I was overjoyed just to be out there pedaling my heart out, day after day.

I think most other parents who had a child with my challenges would have steered their kid away from any kind of athletic activities, but all I wanted to do was to play sports. Fortunately, my parents helped me find a way to do as much as possible within the parameters that hydrocephalus set for me. They taught me to set my own goals and standards. They helped me learn that the way tennis enriched my life was not through blue ribbons or trophies, but through the lifelong friendships I formed, the confidence in my own abilities that I discovered within myself, and the knowledge that doing my personal best within my own unique context was a real and satisfying accomplishment.

My parents taught me to believe in myself. They fostered in me a strong sense of optimism and an excitement about what was possible that helped me tolerate frustration. Their confidence in me helped me to navigate those challenges when a little extra effort was required in order to succeed. They encouraged me to develop a strong internal compass and they honored that, even at times when my endeavors terrified them (the fifteen-hundred-mile bike ride was one of those times).

These incredible gifts that my parents gave me have directly contributed to every success I've enjoyed throughout my life. Ever since my sons were born, I've worked to instill in them the resilience, tenacity, and grace that my parents modeled for me.

The starting horn blew and Alex's boat quickly pulled ahead, leaving the other boats in its wake. John's boat was falling behind, and I watched him struggle to keep up with the other rowers in his boat. He was too far away for me to see the familiar frown of concentration on his face, but I knew it was there. I knew he was giving it everything he had.

A cheer rose from the crowd around me as Alex's boat crossed the finish line. The jubilant boys splashed each other's faces and raised triumphant fists. Once on solid ground, they whooped and hugged each other, along with the friends and family members who had rushed to the shore to congratulate them.

The rest of the boats came to shore soon after. I watched John cross the finish line, his face red with exertion but his smile wide with pride. He made a beeline for his brother, an ecstatic grin plastered across his face.

"You guys did it!" John was saying. "I knew you could!"

All the way home, the two boys sat in the back of the van and talked about how much fun they'd had and how excited they were for the next regatta—how they planned on practicing every chance they got, how much their muscles had grown and would continue to grow...

"Sure, I was hoping we would at least come in second," John said to me later, "but this was only my second regatta. I still have a lot of progress to make." He had done his best and was proud of what he had accomplished.

I'd never seen John so enthusiastic about a sport, and that's saying something because this kid loves sports. "Rowing is my jam," he said. "It doesn't matter whether I'm winning or not."

"You're enjoying the challenge!" I said.

This was a milestone for John. When he was younger, any time he knew he needed to up his game he would get tense and serious, and his nervousness was palpable. Now, the confidence he exuded was breathtaking, and the easygoing assurance with which he approached his rowing practice was making a huge difference. Within a month of that regatta, he improved his time on the rowing machine by ten seconds for two thousand meters—quite a difference!

My parents helped me define my own sphere of normalcy at a time when it seemed like my childhood was anything but normal. They encouraged me to measure my successes within the context of my own experience. I'm deeply grateful to them for these life lessons, and I'm grateful to them all over again as I see my sons learning these lessons as well. They are learning to work with what they've got instead of holding themselves to unrealistic expectations. They are learning to continuously challenge themselves, and to celebrate every time they give their best instead of pinning their hopes on rankings, scores, or any other abstract outcomes.

In my work as a psychologist, performance coach and podcast host, my primary goal is to help those I work with to move through and beyond challenges within their own unique context without ever losing sight of the possibility in front of them. My hope is that after our work together is complete, my clients—whether they are parents, kids, athletes, or entrepreneurs—will believe in themselves more robustly, through helping them to maximize their potential in a way that makes them happy. My intention is similar for those listening to my podcast and I invite you to tune in. Our goal with the show is to ignite a deeper sense of understanding and possibility in moving through challenges while defining our own unique context, building resilience, and maximizing potential.

The challenges we all face in life are real and unavoidable. As long as we maintain a realistic understanding of the unique contexts within which we operate while maintaining a sense of belief and possibility, we can never be defeated.

ABOUT THE AUTHOR

DR. KATE LUND

Dr. Kate Lund is a licensed Clinical Psychologist, Peak Performance Coach, Bestselling Author, and TEDx Speaker.

During Kate's childhood she managed through the challenges of the complex medical condition Hydrocephalus, and as a result, learned at an early age to believe in the possibilities that exist on the other side of challenge.

With specialized training in medical psychology from three hospitals affiliated with Harvard Medical School, she uses a strength and evidence-based approach to help parents and children build resilience so they can thrive in school, sports, and life.

With her TEDx Talk, "Finding the Ordinary within the Extraordinary, the Superpower Children Need," her ongoing podcast, "The Optimized Mind," and her book "Bounce: Help Your Child Build Resilience and Thrive in School, Sports and Life," Kate's on a mission to share the lessons, mindsets, and tools to building more resilience.

Kate is based in Seattle.

CONNECT WITH KATE HERE:

Website: www.katelundspeaks.com

YouTube: https://www.youtube.com/watch?v=-p6YcTsWySU

Book: https://www.amazon.com/Bounce-Resilience-Thrive-School-Sports-ebook/dp/B071YQG6BC

MARGARET MUSCAT

HOW TO ACHIEVE FREEDOM FROM MENTAL CHAOS

TO MENTAL CLARITY AND INNER PEACE

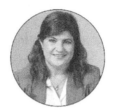

"*W*e all have a cross to bear. We work hard, eat well, and have faith in God." Raised as a Catholic this was the main message I heard as a child, and it impacted most of my life. Self-care and self-love were concepts that were foreign to me.

The first relationship we have is with our parents; they teach and nurture us, doing the best they can. We take all the good, bad, and everything in between, we're the upgraded model, growing up, making a difference in our lives, hoping to be stronger, more resilient, loving, nurturing, happier, wealthier, and better informed.

Whenever anyone suggested a holiday to Malta as beautiful, I struggled to understand or comprehend how. Throughout my life, I heard my parents' painful, hurtful, and traumatising survival stories on repeat. My mom would say "I struggled with the hardship. If you had hardship like I did throughout my life, you wouldn't survive. I am grateful to God that you will never have to suffer hardship and go through what I did." My father would say in his thick Maltese accent "Holidays—it's a waste of time and sports—it's madness, it's danger! They get hurt so let them enjoy it."

My parents grew up in times of manual hard labour, as farmers they used donkeys to pull tillers to turn over soil and grow crops, mum herded sheep, and dad later worked in the mines, later driving trucks. Following their marriage in 1954, they used gelignite to blow up rock, making caves to live in.

Living through the World War in Malta, the most bombed country at that time, mum aged thirteen and dad aged ten, survived war and famine. Humble survivors who succeeded in "all work, no play," they lived a long, hard life still ruminating about their harsh past, preferring to sit and rest, live in peace with gratitude, no lack of food or toiling ever again. They enjoyed eating simple food while they both watched TV. Dad watched the news on television saying, "It's gonna be bad," visited family and relatives, and watched Catholic Mass at home on a video recording played three times a day. There were no hobbies, holidays, and restaurants. Self-worth, self-care, self-love, joy, happiness, celebrating birthdays, Christmas and Easter, having healthy relationships and boundaries, saying "I love you, please and thank you," were non-existent, other than being taught outside our home to be polite and well mannered. Imagine the pressure; my mental health suffered, I internalised the words of my parents, their work ethic, and always put myself last. In this chapter, I share my journey of the impact my parents' beliefs had on me and how I recreated myself, removed the pattern of anxiety, left the past orientation of depression behind, and now am able to help others with their mental health. That's how I make a difference.

I am writing to give you hope because I am definitely not alone in experiencing mental health issues. If I can climb out of the pit of depression and leave the past behind, along with anxious feelings and fear of the unknown—which is anxiety—so can you. At the end, I will give you my favourite tool that has made all the difference in the world in my own healing journey.

BACK TO WHERE IT ALL BEGAN

Dad came to Australia in 1964. Six months later, Mum and eight children joined him as one of the first immigrant families who travelled by airplane. Eight years later they decided to have a "Baby Aussie," a child to look after them for when the other children grew up and left home. I was born their "Baby Kangaroo," their "beautiful little one."

My first language spoken at home was Maltese, so starting school shy and timid, adapting to the English language was challenging. The language at home shaped a very unsocial skillset when I, at sixteen-years-old, and my older siblings ventured out to date and form relationships. Easter eggs and Christmas presents were not given until I had married and had my own four children. Our family worked through all the holidays; it meant working harder on the farm because that's when vegetable prices go up. At age seven I appreciated Uncle Joe taking me to his house to play with my two cousins—we'd also attend church every day during Easter. I missed my parents always, yet going home to my siblings' negative reactions was hard. I knew my parents loved me, even without the words, "I love you," and hugs and kisses, their smiles said it all.

Whenever I had a new toy, my siblings always said, "You're spoiled. You don't deserve that. We never had anything new. We shared everything and everything's secondhand." I told myself, "I wish Mum and Dad would never buy me anything again. I wish my parents would give only to them, so I wouldn't disappoint my siblings ever again." That horrible feeling, not understood as a child, was guilt. The constant language I heard created limiting beliefs, lack of self-confidence, and self-worth, feeling not deserving, negative expectancy, rumination, and inner critic voices that said, "Who would want you? You're not good-looking. You're not good enough." Yet, I wanted someone to love, and to be loved. I just wanted to live a simple life, wanting very little and to be happy. I hoped that "if only," someone would want me, I'd get married, have children, be happy and grateful. Having a career, creating wealth, having choice, being successful were not part of my vocabulary or understanding.

Depression, anxiety, and trauma were my norm, I didn't know about mental health. At sixteen, I expected hardship. Growing up was all work and no play for my siblings, they all pushed each other with demands for assistance and yelled, "Somebody come and bring more boxes," or other requests to get the job done. Conflict started if no one responded, so I became "Somebody" to avoid conflict at all costs. Showing empathy and care to others was so important to me. Survival meant I jumped around quick enough to not get yelled at. I had no voice in a world of watching my siblings argue; the louder they yelled, the less I could speak, and the smaller I became. Respect was given to my parents and to my elders—where did that leave me? People-pleasing was my daily method to cope.

I married young at the age of eighteen. By twenty-eight, I had borne three sons and a daughter, and I couldn't want for more. My Maltese husband was a great provider and my job as a wife was to serve him and care for and raise our children. We were young, raising kids, we never explored how as individuals our relationship with ourselves resulted in mental dysfunction, so our mental health and relationship was destined for failure. *How can you expect to be happy based on a belief that marriage equates to happiness?* The struggle was real. You can create a family, home, car, job, successful business, wealth and not have to struggle in life, yet having all those responsibilities, success, and material things drove me to a deep dark pit of depression. As if I was living in the past of my parents and experiencing their struggle in the present moment, feeling guilty for having it all. I struggled with trying to form relationships for most of my life. Experiencing anxiety and depression together, I asked God, "Why? It shouldn't be this hard, I just want to be happy, I'd give anything just to be happy, to feel normal."

Listening to mass at church, hearing, "It is in giving you shall receive," I gave to my husband, children, parents, and family, yet to myself, I did not believe I was worthy. I experienced overwhelming guilt for having anything good in my life. Putting myself first didn't resonate. Honouring my parents, yes, but honouring myself was selfish. I have since learned and teach my clients that:

To create healthy and loving relationships with others, build your inner self-love first, be kinder to yourself.

How does our environment and the influence of others create and shape our mindset? A negative environment and language, the influence of words heard, create memory retention shaping your inner critic and negative expectancy which affects your internal dialogue. Rumination and negative expectancy in your thought pattern can induce self-criticism resulting in mental exhaustion, leaving you feeling drained, anxious, depressed, and burnt out.

You can't give from an empty cup. Fill your cup first, then you can give and receive love.

Have you witnessed what mental chaos is like? Perhaps you know what it feels like to experience depression and anxiety together? It feels like being in a deep dark pit with no ladder, no light above you, the fear of climbing, to only fall back down stops you before you start. Trying anything and everything to get out of the pit of depression—facing anxiety daily is debilitating.

For twenty-five years the struggle with my mental health continued, finding relief in ways that were short-lived. Counselling felt like getting on and off a merry-go-round, Cognitive Behavioural Therapy was difficult, and imagining a stop sign with a million thoughts running wasn't easy. Constant neck and shoulder pain as a result of bearing the weight of the world on my shoulders from sitting at my desk running the office, physically taking care of home duties, feeling pressure from overexerting my body and mind, keeping on top of motherhood, daily responsibilities as a farmer's wife (meaning he was rarely present to help), and assisting to maintain the heavy load of tasks that ruled me.

Work-life balance creates good mental health, make time!

Following months of treatment from an Osteopath to re-adjust my body, loosen tight muscles and re-align my stiff neck and tense shoulders, he said, "Margaret what are you doing to yourself? You're back to how you were previously. You need to find a solution when it comes to stress! Here's the number of a Hypnotherapist, she will work with you to calm your mind, you can thank me later and this too shall pass." I booked the first appointment; I experienced suicidal thoughts that week and my appointment was brought forward to that afternoon. I recall, "You can lead a horse to water, but you can't make it drink," resonated with me; I wanted to create change, I required to be led to nourish the mind. That day changed me, I was guided to be calm.

A HYPNOTHERAPIST GUIDES YOU TO RELAX THE MIND AND BODY TO CREATE CHANGE, NOT HYPNOTISE YOU!

Hypnotherapy alone helped to create the shift in my mindset by changing my thought process, the negative language of my inner critic, self-worth, and past trauma. By creating a positive expectancy, putting myself first was finally acceptable, not selfish. I no longer experienced that overwhelming feeling of guilt for having success, being deserving and worthy of receiving love, and loving myself through re-creating my identity. Gaining control of my thoughts through hypnotherapy slowed my mind down, I felt better and it enabled me to cope with life. The hypnotherapy journey to climb the mountain began. Reaching the peak, the beauty seen from the top felt like freedom high above the world below. The realization of becoming a Hypnotherapist became my purpose. At the time my husband said that it wasn't possible because of our young family and he needed my support to make our business successful. He said I could study Hypnotherapy once the children left school. I waited twenty years.

I looked for other ways to fulfill my purpose. I found a volunteer association called MIEA (Mental Illness Education Australia) and volunteered to present and educate at secondary schools, teaching the five mental health disorders, how to reach out for help and support a loved one experiencing mental health issues, also sharing my story and experience of depression and anxiety. After one of the presentations, a teacher approached me and said, "Margaret, we can't thank you enough for sharing your story. Because of you, that girl in the front row, who we have been trying to get to speak to the school counsellor for months, finally reached out today." That day, I *Made A Difference*.

The continued responsibility of running a business and lack of time prevented me from playing sports. The old thought pattern, my father's strong words, "It's danger," changed with hypnosis to create new beliefs about physical activity. Nourishing the mind *and* body is important and I recognized that with my mind in a better space, it was time to focus on my body to strengthen myself physically. Knowing exercise also benefits mental health, I started to play soccer—and continued to do so for six years. It became part of my self-care routine. Getting my body fit and mobile again was an outlet to feel freedom and release the frustrations of debtors and countless hours of sitting behind a desk. After a major fall that injured my jaw, I chose to quit soccer. I couldn't risk reinjuring myself as I was in constant pain with my jaw for the next few years. Not playing soccer and jaw pain affected my mental health.

Stress and depression followed after quitting soccer, and my psychiatrist prescribed medication to treat the anxiety and depression. The medication left me feeling numb, like I was not present, and six-years later the medication stopped working. Acupuncture felt good for a few days after treatment until I experienced a nervous breakdown as the financial stress and responsibility led me into a downward spiral. I looked up Electroconvulsive Therapy because I was desperate for relief. My psychiatrist refused me ECT treatment, he suggested hospitalisation and receiving medical treatment there. Hospitalization, I felt, was admitting failure.

I decided to relax at home; my belief was that resting and caring for myself alone in my safe place would be most beneficial. Medication changes and the increased doses did not help and created frustration. A clinical trial was advertised. The study investigated Ketamine, an anesthetic drug used to treat survivors from active war zones suffering Post Traumatic Stress Disorder that could also treat severe depression. I participated in the trial, and the Ketamine injections worked amazing for me right up until the trial clinic was shut down six months later.

Why is physical activity so important to having good Mental Health? Exercise releases chemicals like endorphins and serotonin that improve your mood. Take time out to recharge your body and clear your thoughts, get physical, make walking a part of your mental health self-care routine. Team sports build confidence, social skills, and teamwork aids as an outlet for releasing daily stress and creating a healthy work-life balance.

Take time out, build, manage and maintain your mental health through exercise and self-care!

Ready to pursue my dream, I studied Clinical Hypnotherapy and Strategic Psychotherapy, Hypnosis, Neuro-Linguistic Programming (NLP), and Time-Line Based Therapy. I began investing in myself. No longer suppressing my purpose to help others with years of knowledge I'd experienced finally came to fruition! I found the name "Gordon Young" in a note given to me by Rae, my hypnotherapist, twenty years ago, to find he *is* the founder of the Institute of Applied Psychology. I attended a seminar and registered that night with my husband present. He said, "I don't think this is a good idea and it's costly." My response was "I'm going to do this, with or without your approval."

At forty-six years of age, "Maltese farm girl and businesswoman" began training for a career in Mental Health. Despite thoughts and expectations of failure, *I passed!* In training, I was Gordon's ideal client and often he used me as an example in teaching. The words in hypnosis that resonated most were, "Leave behind anything which no longer serves you, and bring with you any resources into the present," and, "Negative words and thoughts don't stick, they slide right off you, you're like Teflon." Respect for myself was found in practical sessions throughout the courses; I'd never had respect for myself so finding the strength to say, "No," and serving myself without feeling selfish or guilty was life-changing. Now I'm able to give back to the world, the time has arrived to give the best version of myself.

I was ready to take control of my life, to "be kinder to myself," to create my identity, the "Margaret of the future," where the possibilities are endless. A life I had never imagined—*freedom* from anxiety and depression for good. *Letting Go* of the remaining limiting beliefs that no longer served me, and to build my self-worth to heights not reached previously. Believing that, "You're going to be an amazing Hypnotherapist Margaret," as I was told by Rae twenty-years earlier, became a reality.

My positive attitude grew stronger within me and continued to change. Close relationships also started to change and some broke down, as a result of respecting myself.

Saying "no" to pleasing people is empowering.

Living in a money-driven world, not purpose-driven, and being immersed in the toxic environment of negative attitudes, I realised staying in the surrounding environment and maintaining good mental health wasn't possible. Fearing the word "divorce," I chose "separation," and ended my marriage of twenty-eight years. *Letting Go* of those I loved who did not support my choices and newfound happiness, to have *Mental Clarity and Inner Peace*. Letting go of the life, family, and business built over thirty-years was my greatest fear. I was misunderstood, being told, "You're being selfish," "You've changed," and "We don't know who you are anymore." Even after passing my three diplomas, I was told, "You need help, go see a therapist."

We must be willing to Let Go of the life we had planned, to accept the one that is waiting for us.

I spent time alone, being grateful for the past lessons, knowing the strength it would take to survive this journey alone with family conflict all around me, comforting myself. I created healthy boundaries in relationships, saying, "No," to disrespect. Arguing was no point, attempting to justify my decisions. I was no longer being referred to as "Somebody," now I'm me, "*just*, Margaret." I believe in myself, and I know my worth. With my daughter, Christine, and my best friend, Rose, by my side, I met Mark, my partner, five months after separating, also making new friends who became family and supported me. The healing journey and experience over the next two years led me to begin my business: *Hilltop Hypnotherapy—"When life changes to be harder, change yourself to be stronger."*

To create mental clarity and inner peace, be open to suggestions through hypnotherapy.

The *Journey to Make A Difference* by guiding clients to better mental health using Strategic Psychotherapy to find their resources and bring them back to the present, and using hypnosis in a relaxed environment. Clients take back control of their vehicle called life, breaking free from fearing the unforeseeable future as anxiety, and leaving the past emotion attached with depression behind them. They quit "self-soothing anxiety" or "trauma with addictions," and remove the emotional entrapment associated with Complex Post Traumatic Stress Disorder (CPTSD) using NLP dissociation techniques through absurdity, to detach the emotional links from trauma, achieving *Freedom!*

My goal in life is to guide my clients to achieve control of their lives, and create mental clarity, freedom, happiness, inner peace, and joy, as I have. *To LIVE, LAUGH AND LOVE LIFE as, Who I Am—"Margaret."*

ABOUT THE AUTHOR

MARGARET MUSCAT

Margaret Muscat CHT. is the Founder of Hilltop Hypnotherapy. In 2018, she obtained a Diploma in Strategic Psychotherapy and Hypnosis, Practitioner of Neuro Linguistic Programming (NLP), and Practitioner of Time-line Based Therapy.

Using Strategic Psychotherapy to determine the client's resources and using Hypnosis to break limiting beliefs and unhealthy patterns, she treats Mental Health clients presenting with Anxiety, Depression, PTSD, Insomnia and Self-Esteem, and Addictions such as Alcohol & Gambling. Margaret creates resourceful, happier, healthier mindset in her clients within a relaxed environment that allows mental clarity.

Raised as the daughter of a vegetable farmer in Hawkesbury, Sydney NSW, Margaret then married in 1990 and raised four children whilst farming turf/sod, in 2008 owning and operating as Company Director and Secretary, Accounts Manager in Turf Production Sales and Marketing. In 2003, she volunteered at MIEA as Mental Health Educator and Presenter in secondary Schools. Her leading Agribusiness won the Local Outstanding Agricultural Business Award in 2012, and Champion Agribusiness in the Australian Small Business Awards 2013.

Margaret now lives with her partner, Mark, in Mulgoa, NSW and is proud to achieve her dream of becoming an author in 2023.

CONNECT WITH MARGARET HERE:

Website: https://www.hilltophypnotherapy.com.au/

Free Gift: Relaxation to Mental Clarity and Inner Peace (Audio Recording)

For all socials and link to gift: http://linktr.ee/margaretmuscat

LAILA ANSARI

DITCH THE SCRIPT

LIFE IS AN IMPROV

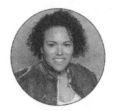

*I*t was the summer of 2016. We were deep in conversation.

Although I hadn't seen my girlfriend for a while, I loved our impromptu catch-ups which usually involved eating delicious food accompanied by raucous laughter and chitter-chatter about nothing and everything under the sun. Suddenly, I was triggered by something she said and I could feel my mood wane into deep thoughts. I quickly readjusted my focus on our gathering and returned to our discussion. You see, my friend was taking an improvisation course and I was intrigued by the material and elements she was sharing over our meal. I wanted to know more about where and how to join a similar course. That's when she said, "You don't need an improv course, your entire life is an improv."

At that moment, we both laughed it off, finished our meal and happily departed to go about our business. But my mind was still hanging on to her words; they stuck with me for days, playing over and over again in my head.

What did she mean?

Was that a compliment or was she poking fun at me?

How was my life an improv?

And how was I not even aware of it?

I was left perplexed while also curious about what that could mean. It took a long time for me to realise the treasure she saw within me on that day, a treasure I had never, until that moment, seen within myself.

I had always thought I was struggling through life with no clear plan, grasping every opportunity that came my way, secretly low in self-esteem, and believing that I could not actually have what I wanted. But when she put it to me like that, I realised she did mean it as a compliment. In all my "improvisations" I had developed the skill to duck the punches life threw at me and, somehow, always find a way around the obstacles to make it out of any situation alive and on top.

Let me explain.

Here I was, fresh out of college, very eager to leave student life behind and forge a successful career ahead of me as an Early Childhood teacher. The hard work had come to an end for the moment, and I felt it was time to celebrate and spread my wings!

Living independently in London as a young Black American woman in a city with a population of nearly seven million, I loved the bustling streets with their red, open-backed double-decker buses, the densely built cobble-stoned roads lined with modern and ancient buildings all crammed together, and street after street teeming with people from everywhere. The air was electrifying, I could not help but feel the surge of energy and vibration thrusting me into its swarm, feelings that everyone had somewhere to go or something to do! Their "doing" seemed to be full of focus and purpose. For me, London was both exciting and overwhelming all at once.

On one hand, the city was full of opportunities for growth, self-discovery, and exploration, with its countless cultural events, spectacular historical sights, galleries, museums, nightlife, food from every corner of the world, and entertainment to cater for all kinds of people. On the other hand, it could be a place of deep loneliness, struggle, and intimidation, along with many cunning and manipulative individuals who were looking to prey on naïve, vulnerable, and kind-hearted people. It took some time to adjust to navigating around this cosmopolitan city and assimilate to the vast cultural differences despite speaking the same language. Little did I know that I would need to physically hustle and lean on my years of improv as a child and adolescent to continue to enjoy my newfound freedoms while struggling to survive, thrive, and succeed in this city of no mercy.

I felt like I was a good person because I came from a good family, even though my parents were authoritarian in the way they raised us. My upbringing had been somewhat like living in a pressure cooker; being the eldest of five children, I had been handed the role of matriarch for my younger siblings. Should anything happen to them, I was held hugely responsible. As a child, I had to figure out a way to survive that pressure and learn to be quick-witted, a problem solver, and read situations and people intuitively. That is how I began my life of improv without even realising—I had to be everything to everyone and think on my feet to see how I could manage the demands of all those roles. Through my program of survival, I ultimately lost who I was by becoming the caretaker of those around me. That became my mission in life and what I was "good" at, without even realising it was at my own expense.

People tended to label me from early on and put me into boxes. Many of those boxes were not positive, which made me feel small and misunderstood, and reinforced and negatively imprinted on my internal beliefs about myself. Because I came across as a confident, resourceful, natural leader, I was always blamed whenever the children got into trouble. Instead, the adults looked at me and said, "Jeez you're precocious." I was often called "sassy," "fast," and even "divisive." My understanding was they weren't being kind and I wanted to know what made them not like me.

Because I didn't know how to play the game of approval and praise with the big people, beneath the surface my mental state was insecure and uncertain. My point of view was always, "She's better than me, she's smarter or prettier," or, "They come from a better background or family," and the big one, "Those types of things don't happen to me." And so, they never did. I never knew why either, other than what I made up in my head. I just knew I wasn't lucky.

I was heartbroken many times. Spending days and nights crying my eyeballs out behind closed doors. When a guy didn't choose to be with me, I'd be devastated. When the job opportunity didn't come my way, I became resentful which often caused me to leave my job or end up being dismissed. This vicious circle left me feeling like I wasn't worthy or good enough. Nevertheless, I woke up every day and started all over again, being the performer in my head! Lights. Camera. Action. I would put on that mask, the hat, whatever it took to get through the days, while leaving my soul and essence behind—because that part of me was too cut up and raw to showcase to the world. Not realising that this was the most crucial ingredient and the key to my being! My sparkle, my spirit! No amount of great improvisation on my part was ever fully received by anyone, no matter where I went or whatever I was attempting to obtain, because my heart and soul weren't in it. Without me embodying my complete self, no one of real worth, influence, and power was buying into me.

But as time passed, it took me longer and longer to get back on my feet whenever life threw me a curveball. The performer was growing weary, and I didn't even realise it.

After some time floating around in meaningless jobs, simply to make ends meet, while still feeling misunderstood, my attention seemed to pivot towards testing and measuring which man could be the key to my salvation and happiness. At that point, happiness didn't live within me without having someone else to be the catalyst for the creation of happiness. When I was alone, my demons would surface and pick at me, opening scar tissue and unhealed wounds. Being with someone else enabled me to suppress my loathsomeness towards myself and made me feel liked, loved, and appreciated for all the things I could do for them to show my worthiness. On the days when I allowed my mind to tear me to shreds, I would chant to myself, "Life is to give and not to take," totally missing out on the fact that I never allowed myself to keep anything back for myself. All I knew was 'to give, give, give, and give some more.'

Looking back on that journey now, I was married to a beautiful man who, I believed, loved me to death, yet the relationship was doomed from the start. It was doomed because I didn't know how to create joy, happiness, stability, and abundance from within me and me alone. All my feelings and actions were fixated externally. During that time, I projected "everything I wasn't" onto my husband and everyone else in an attempt to make it their problem too. And the crazy thing is, I was completely unaware of my own manipulation and self-sabotage.

What I really needed was to cultivate a good sense of my own purpose, based upon my beliefs, values, and a true, deep connection within myself. There was no script or pre-planned dialogue I could prepare, despite so desperately wanting one. As with any show, I had to be open and receptive to whatever came my way, and trust in my instincts to guide me towards the right decisions for myself based on notes from my past lessons.

For many years, I surrendered to not knowing what I should do, or be, in this life. I tried my hand at many different careers, interests and skills, but none of them gave me internal fulfilment. Despite it all, I never gave up on stoking the fire of my internal desire to ask, "Where do I *make a difference* for myself and the ones I hold dear to me?" Then, in what seemed like in an instant, on one given day I wasn't seeking the answer anymore. I am now four years into being a professional Motivational Speaker and Relationship Coach.

At that moment during lunch with my friend, something inside me was awakened by our random conversation, which then caused a cascade of unconscious decisions that led me to my "unicorn job" in helping others. The irony is that I have always loved to help others around me but I didn't understand the importance of helping myself first, to then have the positive outcome I sought for those who came into my life.

The *journey back to myself* has been a double-edged sword. Many times I wanted to quit, and I did attempt to quit by sometimes allowing myself to stagnate for days and weeks on end. But the yearning for something else much greater than the existing pain I had settled with for decades didn't feel the same. A new sensation was growing within me, calling me to embrace my fears and everything else I had been carrying for far too long. As a result I began to clean out my closet of historical emotional baggage.

My current work is beyond anything I have imagined. In helping other professional women find deeper love within themselves so they can share this with someone else, I have also strengthened who I am. I truly see and know we are not alone in this journey, no matter how alone we may feel at any given moment. And when we look through the lens of our inner light and beauty, we see so many precious gems sprinkled along our path. These gems light up and reflect as we grow trust within, that then illuminates and amplifies our greatness and importance through self-love and acceptance. When this starts to take hold, it creates a ripple effect and chain reaction in all aspects of our life—and more positive possibilities come our way.

I have identified four steps that elevated me further in my personal growth to become who I am today. When you live in a place of certainty that you, and you alone, have control over how you see things in life—which shapes how you react to situations and promotes how you behave and interact with others—you can steer your life's journey with your head held high, feeling proud of who you are and where you are going.

Here I share with you the core fundamentals, so you too can become the best version of you. They will help you begin to identify which step along your journey you have arrived at and need to take a closer look.

1. SELF-AWARENESS

The first step in my journey of transformation was *self-awareness*. I had to stop looking away from myself to find the reason my life was not the way I wanted it to be. Instead, I had to slowly recognise the positive things I was achieving and the wonderful perceptions others had about me. I also needed to acknowledge that my role, my behaviour, and my thinking was keeping me stuck in the same situation, time and time again. I had to confront the negative self-talk I so faithfully spent years nurturing and growing like a farmer in their field, going out daily to ensure their crops will come to harvest. I, too, had become very good at beating myself up on a grand scale and I needed to tell myself, sometimes even out loud, to *"Shut up! Please, just shut up!"* It was necessary to stop the negative talk that cultivated my limiting beliefs and ensured my actions of self-sabotage and comparing myself to any others who were a fraction better than me. My God! It was not an easy process but I held on to the belief I would change for the better and over time, the universe sent me challenges to show me the work I had done was not in vain.

2. OWNERSHIP

Next, I had to take *ownership* for my actions and the outcome of the decisions I was making. Oh man. How hard is it to stare down the barrel of your own mess and throw your arms in the air, professing, it was, "all you and no one else!" Ouch. That was an even bigger mountain to climb and overcome. Getting through it was so liberating and empowering once I wasn't standing neck deep in my own blame game. Instead of seeing myself as a victim of circumstances, like in the past, I began to see myself as a human who makes mistakes but can learn from them and overcome my challenge and come out better. This meant my setbacks weren't so dramatic and damning, and I also didn't need to retreat into hiding, thinking that everyone also thought I was a "loser." Over time, my luck started to change and there were more positive things coming my way. With it also came positive and encouraging people to help me lift my game even more. The need to feel validated, accepted, and care about the opinions of others grew less. And with this too, I felt a new sense of control of my life, and happiness within me that I had not felt for a very long time.

3. INTEGRITY AND SELF-DISCIPLINE

Another important aspect of this transformation was to act on the things I said I valued. For a long time I was not reliable which negatively impacted my relationships with others and my work ethic. I wanted to be consistent in my behaviour because sometimes I was reliable, and other times I allowed what was going on to give me an excuse to not show up to my commitments. This could cause conflict and also damage my reputation as an honest, reliable person of integrity. I said I was those things, but my behaviour undermined my values. Hard work was needed to ensure what I said I valued and how I demonstrated this were aligned and congruent with who I was being. Learning to be the trustworthy person I thought I was meant becoming more self-disciplined with myself, for myself, and towards others. This required me to stop playing out my old patterns and reactions when things were not going according to my old script, and choosing to lean into my zone of discomfort with openness and positivity.

82

4. SELF-COMPASSION

Perhaps the most significant shift of all occurred when I realised my true fulfilment and happiness could only come from within. For decades, I spent time perfecting how to limit my horizons and play out my life, feeling small. My life was not a tragedy. I lived a life many would envy from the outside and I taught myself to accept what I was given and to be grateful for what I had. But during that conversation with my girlfriend many moons ago, my subconscious was stirred, leading me to discover my treasure trove hidden inside me. I now know I had been following a script others had written for me and it was time for me to embrace the uncertainty of my own unwritten script so I could create my own story, on my own terms. I needed to forgive myself and let go of this notion that because I wasn't doing life "perfectly," I wasn't allowed to "level up" and dream big. Until that moment during lunch, I looked up to my girlfriend as being "the person who had everything" and I felt so privileged that she found me interesting. My gratitude towards this moment in time is boundless because I chose to listen to my inner calling and fall into the unknown within that had been hidden from me. Now, I show up daily with self-compassion and determination in knowing *I am enough*.

I repeatedly acknowledge my strengths from within that enable me to develop the resilience needed in the face of adversity. The adversities I have experienced throughout my life have aided in my resilience and enabled me to be the adaptable person I am today. I happily acknowledge this as one of my strengths. Arriving at the feeling of being whole has given me such beautiful peace. I gave myself no "out" on the baptism of fire, but chose to throw myself into the flames of my known existence with the confidence and certainty that when I came out the other side, I would be a better person. This experience gave me a huge dose of learning how to be self-compassionate, and to show myself forgiveness for all the poor decisions and mistakes I made over the years. My failures and reckless choices all are woven into the tapestry of who I am. I no longer lament my battle scars from life, for they are a vast part of my beauty and the richness I bring to this life and those I choose to show up for. I always remember to start with me.

The adversity we all feel is called life. Find the treasure hidden deep within you to lift your spirit and help raise your vibration for a better you. Your biggest unused resource is acknowledging that you have no script! So let go of trying to create one. Embrace life as an improv, where you have the power to create your own story. Believe in yourself, take ownership of your life, and be kind to yourself along the way. Know you are capable of anything once you make the decision. And remember—you are not a victim of your circumstances and they do not define you or your future.

"You may encounter many defeats, but you must not be defeated. In fact, it may be necessary to encounter the defeats, so you can know who you are, what you can rise from, how you can still come out of it."
-Maya Angelou

ABOUT THE AUTHOR

LAILA ANSARI

Laila Ansari is an Amazon Bestselling Author, Motivational Speaker, and Relationship Coach who is renowned for being a "life and people lover" to all she meets.

She has dedicated her career to helping individuals achieve a deeper connection and understanding of themselves.

Raised in California, Laila grew up in a multicultural environment that fostered her interest in human behavior and psychology. Laila has spent many years in an HR capacity in the commercial sector and as a business owner, which led her on the journey of exploration into the field of Life Coaching. She is an NLP Practitioner and has avidly studied Positive Psychology, Meta programs and Family Systems.

Laila is passionate about sharing the importance of "Self Love" with the world through storytelling about resilience, courage, compassion and forgiveness.

CONNECT WITH LAILA HERE:

Website: https://www.lailaansari.com/

Free Gift: https://lailaansari.com/relationship-e-book

For all socials and podcast: https://linktr.ee/lailaansari

ANDREW DE SOUZA

"VUCA IS NOW VUCAP!"

EMBRACING POLARITY IN AN EVER-CONTENTIOUS WORLD

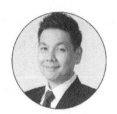

I was at the conclusion of a two-year-long research that spanned across the first primary years of the COVID-19 pandemic. At that point of time, my imposter syndrome set in as I considered adding an additional letter to an acronym that has been known for almost thirty-five years: VUCA.

The term VUCA, based on the leadership theories of economists and university professors Warren Bennis and Burt Nanus, has long been accepted and widely used to describe the Volatile, Uncertain, Complex, and Ambiguous environment of the world we live in. I thought it was ridiculous and questioned myself over who I thought I was to be audaciously adding another letter to this well-established acronym. I did it anyway! I penned it down as one of the key concluding statements in my doctorate thesis in Business Administration.

VUCA is now VUCAP!

Even for those who have never heard of VUCA previously, the COVID-19 pandemic would have given anyone first-hand experience of at least one of the four situations. One would then wonder why there is a need to discuss VUCA again, given the fact that we already had a taste of it across the past few years. Well, the focus was never about VUCA. Instead, it is about adding the letter 'P' to describe how polarized or polarizing the world has become. Bear with me as I explain why this is important.

P FOR POLARIZED / POLARITY

In the course of my work, I am approached by my peers and clients for advice on a diverse area of matters. While most of it revolves around the domain of business management and taxation, I am also consulted on matters that are more personal. I have been told my analytical ability allows me to provide different perspectives which, in turn, help uncover potential pitfalls that most may not see at first. However, this clear-headedness of mine vaporizes the moment I am enraged. This happens whenever I am in disagreement. My wife, who is a crucial support pillar to me, is regularly entertained by my anger management challenges. This makes the topic of polarity something meaningful that I want to share.

Polarity, a word that is more commonly used in science, defines a state of complete opposites. In my context, I am using it to describe having opposing views, beliefs, or opinions on any subject or matter. These differences, if not handled carefully, can cause rage or fuel conflict. While this is an account from my own observations, I believe we will have to address this sooner rather than later. Coining this new term VUCAP is my attempt to draw your attention to an ever-changing and contentious world, and arming us with understanding and tools on how to bridge the divides is how I intend to make a difference.

Will our differences make us better or will they tear us apart?

As a tenured member of a business community for thirteen years, I have abided by the unspoken rule of avoiding certain sensitive topics in my usual conversations with fellow members. Topics such as gender, racial, religious, and political discussions can evoke strong emotions that affect the social fabric of the community. Back at home, my dad and I shared very polarized views when it came to politics and we never seemed to end any political discussion amicably. To make matters worse, we now live in the digital age where our vast and easy access to information from new media grants us the liberty to adopt different opinions or even develop new ones of our own. These differing opinions can be so contrasting that they constantly create new divides.

NOT JUST ANOTHER LESSON FROM COVID-19

Last year, as I started to pay closer attention to the online and offline conversations of my peers, I arrived at a discovery that there was a rising number of issues that people disagree on. Such issues have gone beyond the commonly avoided topics of gender, race, religion and politics. As the perpetual educator, the COVID-19 pandemic opened my eyes to this interesting realization. Back at that time, I found people disagreeing on issues created by COVID-19. Examples include the debate on whether vaccination was safe, whether borders should remain shut or reopened, and whether the workforce should continue to work remotely or return to office. With the pandemic now being more or less over, most of these issues are no longer as noteworthy as before. Yet we have to remember that once upon a time, these issues polarized people to the point where almost no foreseeable compromise or middle ground could be reached.

A more recent case that is fresh in my mind is from the gaming industry. This year, one of the games I have played since childhood is releasing a fourth edition of its series. It is one of the most highly anticipated releases happening of 2023. Gone are the days when it was a simpler process for games in which the publisher dictates most of the game design. Gamers were handed just a take-it-or-leave-it approach; if they liked what was made, they could continue playing, otherwise choose something else. What we are now experiencing for a new game, that is less than a month from its official release, is a community divided on how the game should be moving forward. With the vast number of enthusiasts sharing their opinions over social media and video sharing platforms, I cannot imagine how challenging it is to be a game publisher these days. Having to strike a balance between creating something enticingly unique while juggling the need to appease the community of fans at large, one small misstep could lead to a fury of zero-star reviews across all ratings platforms.

MITIGATING THROUGH THE POLARIZED WORLD: LET'S START WITH AWARENESS

How should we deal with this increasingly polarizing world? I believe it all starts with raising awareness on the matter. Back in 2022 when this first caught my attention, I started becoming more sensitive and began observing the discordances around me. This heightened level of awareness brought about a motivation to address the issue head on and think of solutions. As a result, I arrived at three possible ways to move forward.

APPROACH 1 - AVOIDANCE

The first way forward was to continue adopting the cautious approach of not engaging in any conversations or debates on topics that evoke strong emotions. Avoidance is the art of choosing our battles; not all battles are worth engaging in. I couldn't find a better way to illustrate this point than by sharing this memorable lesson I got from my officer-in-charge during the final interview just days before I left the military. This officer often regarded himself as a "farmer," a term commonly used in the military to describe soldiers who rely more on brawn over brains. Uncharacteristically, he shared the following ideology about war, battles, and peace, "In a war, there are many battles and we always want to win as many battles as possible. However, a war is not won by winning every battle, a war is won when peace is attained." In this increasingly polarized world, avoiding potential conflict by choosing our battles carefully might indeed be a wiser choice. Hence, before engaging in any debate, it would be useful to first assess whether this is a battle worth fighting for.

APPROACH 2 - ATTRACTION

The second way forward adopts a more proactive approach to take a stand. It draws the principles from the Law of Attraction. Just as like attracts like, great minds think alike and birds of the same feather flock together. If we take some time off to evaluate the people around us—our peers, colleagues or even customers—we will often realize that we tend to attract people who share similar beliefs and values to us. While the first approach was to adopt a passive stance, we may find ourselves in situations where we have to take an active stance. When a time like that arises, standing firm to what we truly believe in enables us to attract like-minded individuals. If we are to adopt this approach, we need to know that we will never be able to please every single person out there. We will attract our loyal supporters and offend our haters. Rather than trying to convince or compromise with someone having contrasting beliefs, wouldn't it be easier to work with those who share the same beliefs as us?

APPROACH 3 - ACCEPTANCE

The third and final way forward is to reach an acceptance. As I get wiser, I have learned to appreciate this approach much more. While I initially argued that none of the three approaches were superior to the other, I came to realize that the other two fuel some form of conflict either internally or externally. If we ever arrive at a level of acceptance we can, in fact, escape the divisive comportments and create harmony in an environment of diverse views. This, unfortunately, is easier said than done. What I can offer is three simple steps which I have termed "OEM" along with some personal examples to show you how I am paving my way to reaching this acceptance.

O: Be Open-minded

Being open-minded is about denoting receptivity to newer ideas or views. Exposing ourselves, or acknowledging differing points of view, does not equate to an agreement. We can always listen with an open heart and mind without needing to agree. Furthermore, we can still be kind even if we disagree. There isn't a need to put anyone down in shame or in a position of disempowerment for persevering with their views. My friend Charlie subscribes to some of the most controversial theories with regards to the topic of vaccination. I always feel very entertained whenever he shares these theories with us, although I find it hard to accept them as I am on the other end of the spectrum. Charlie left his high-paying job in the middle of the pandemic when his company imposed a mandatory vaccination policy. While I will never be able to agree with Charlie, I do respect him for the sacrifice he made and sticking firm to his beliefs.

E: Be Empathetic

Just like the example of Charlie, sometimes we have to dig deeper to find out the underlying reasons why a particular person may have strong views on a topic or subject matter. A close friend of mine, Douglas, who is an affable and good-natured person, almost overnight turned very vocal when discussions were happening about the reopening of borders. He regularly posted harsh comments on social media that criticized the overly cautious approach taken by the authorities to defer the reopening of borders. Some of my peers, including myself, initially found him to be a nuisance. However, upon understanding the struggles he was experiencing at home, we were able to empathize with him. Douglas' dad was terminally ill and he was desperately in need of a medically-trained helper to provide palliative care. The border closures resulted in a shortage and he was losing patience with the authorities. Everyone has a hidden story. Learning to see beyond the surface empathically could help us be more patient and accommodating towards people with differing views.

M: Be Mindful

My definition of mindfulness here is about developing a deeper level of awareness to reach the stage of acceptance, without being overly reactive or overwhelmed by what's going on. I won't be surprised if you have an entirely different definition for the term mindfulness. A recent incident taught us that deliberating about differing definitions can often be a pointless process. A Singaporean girl was mocked mercilessly on the internet after labeling a bag from a local fashion retailer as a luxury item. In view of her family's humble financial situation, the gift she received from her father meant a lot to her and it was a devastating experience to be on the receiving end of such hate. Contrary to the common belief, not every argument or debate has to end with an outcome, or at least reach a middle ground. Times have changed and we should start to accept the fact that reaching the middle ground is no longer mandatory. Considering how inconclusive some present-day debates can be, this middle ground could in fact be non-existent. We should instead adopt the alternative notion of agreeing to disagree.

Will VUCAP ever be the accepted acronym? I certainly don't know. The truth remains that the world is definitely getting more polarized as we speak. The sooner we come to terms with it, the sooner we can start to figure out how we, as individuals, leaders, and even businesses can brace ourselves for this polarization, just as we have learned to embrace VUCA.

If you ever find yourself in a polarized situation, I hope the above approaches will be helpful in guiding you to mitigate conflict and emerge as a stronger person.

ABOUT THE AUTHOR

ANDREW DE SOUZA

Inspired by the quote, "Pray not that you don't die, but that you don't die without having fully lived and loved," Andrew de Souza aspires to uplift more people to overcome their obstacles and live a fulfilling life.

He is the Co-Founder of Regenesis Global, a mission-driven company that focuses on helping aspiring individuals achieve self-transformation and start their journey as an entrepreneur. Perhaps surprisingly, he has a background as a Tax Practitioner who has helped multiple businesses mitigate complex matters in taxation and compliance.

Andrew is often sought after as a fourth-generation action-learning practitioner for his insights, wisdom, and problem-solving ability. He is highly regarded as a notorious networker in the entrepreneurial business community and was awarded a Doctorate in Business Administration for his thesis on driving performance in business communities with ©Project-Based Accelerated Action Learning.

Andrew is based in Singapore with his lovely wife and son.

CONNECT WITH ANDREW HERE:

For all socials: https://linktr.ee/andesouza

DEENA SYED

ROAD TO REDEMPTION

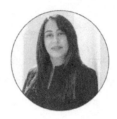

*A*s I stared outside the fourteenth floor window into the grey sky of

Ganzhou, I felt numb and lonely. My dream career had become a nightmare. *What am I doing in a city where the sky is always grey and the people work like robots to make things worth nothing? Is this what I have worked so hard for the past fifteen years? For the "Greed economy," marketing cheap products for an insatiable consumerist society?*

All these thoughts ran through my mind in a split second and I felt like a fraud. Like so many colleagues, I was constantly striving for wins, fame, and titles. Prestigious business trips, designer bags, impressive shoes, fancy restaurants, power plays in boardrooms. Winning at all costs made me the ultimate survivor, but little did I know how my soul was being crushed. Not being able to feel my heart anymore. Not recognisable to my family and old friends. I felt empty under layers of expensive clothing, a façade of strength on my face. That resting bitch face that I learnt to master over the years to control people around me. This was the realisation that I had lost the sense of who I was.

THE RE-DISCOVERY OF ME

Too distraught to return to work after another red-eye flight, I called in sick. This was something I only did when I burnt myself out; usually, I would fly back at 1 am and still be in the office by 9 am sharp, still high from the trip. But this time I was feeling depressed and couldn't pretend anymore that my career was so important to me. After all, it nearly cost me my family. I was estranged from them because I did not have time for myself, or for them. I was consumed by the desire to achieve more and more. So, in the next few months, I phased myself out of my job.

Great at self-sabotage, especially when resentful—and I resented who I had become—I began to show the directors that they didn't need me. In proving this, not only was I extremely disagreeable and disruptive to the executive team, but I also started to create new processes to help the team manage the day-to-day marketing activities without my input. Let's face it, I had lost interest and could no longer pretend. Soon enough, the desire to dress up as a power bitch was fading and I was letting myself go. It was time to leave and find the meaning in my life.

Unexpectedly, the idea of leaving work brought a lot of joy to my family. They saw how much work distracted me but never discouraged me from pursuing my ambitions. I took time off to bond with my family, heal my burnt-out body and look for my passions and new opportunities. Little did I know that I was opening a can of worms. When you lose the one status you worked so hard for, you feel worthless and realise how labels were holding you captive.

Now that I was no longer the Head of Marketing, what was I? A mum? A house-wife? A woman? I felt like I was nothing. This was not something I was used to. Being overly busy with life at home and work was my escape. It was a way to avoid self-reflection and ponder the hard questions that sometimes surface. Now there was no escape and I had to face the fact that I didn't know who I was, what I wanted out of life, and what God wanted from me. "This must be what they call an existential crisis," I thought in my darkest reflections. Not wanting to share my feelings with anyone (after all, I was this flawless ideal I had created), I decided to find a way out of it myself. I decided to focus on what I didn't like about what I'd become.

Being overweight and fatigued was the first thing that stood out. So, it was time to de-stress, detox, and declutter. I started a new Keto diet to address some of my adrenal issues. With the support of my naturopath, I started intermittent fasting and within six months, I lost over ten unwanted kilos. I ditched sugar, which reversed my hypothyroidism and I became much clearer in my mind. When you cut out sugar and processed food, you start experiencing sweetness in everything; even a single lettuce leaf is like a dessert.

Fascinated by the fact that I was feeling the world around me again, I started to explore other sensory experiences through *Qi Gong* and sound frequencies. Over the years, I had tried various modalities to relax and de-stress, but never fully immersed myself in any of them. This time, my body was healing and my mind was open.

My clothes didn't fit me anymore. Since I did not want to return to the corporate world, these power suits, lavish designer bags, and pointy leather heels were no longer aligned with me. So they all had to go. But this meant letting go, which was inconceivable for a control freak. As I swapped the fitted clothes for loose jumpsuits and hung out with more free-thinking friends, the walls collapsed to reveal a more content version of me. A version that was not so preoccupied with perfection. My creativity surged as my friendships blossomed, and life was not a race anymore. Things and people started flowing to me.

NO CHOICE BUT TO SURRENDER

Flow was a new word in my vocabulary. I was a control freak who realised she had no control over anything. The funny thing was that as I surrendered to life and stopped planning rigorously, I felt that God was planning for me instead. I started to observe the phenomena of synchronicity. Out of the blue, a business acquaintance I hadn't seen in ten years reached out to me to offer a role as a circle leader in an acclaimed networking group in Perth. Friends started to send me the details of business owners who needed marketing help. And, just like that, I became a marketing consultant and the money flowed in.

As this "state of flow" seemed to work well, I was determined to stick to it. Surrendering was a choice that soon became an asset as we were suddenly thrown into an unpredictable worldwide lockdown. I was fortunate to have grown to know myself before the Covid crisis, as the old me wouldn't have been able to cope with confinement. The new me was still finding it hard, but instead of fighting the circumstances, I was aware, awake, and alert. There was no place for denial in this experience. Fear of running out of money, and losing our freedom and basic human rights were everywhere.

I was blessed to have a strong support group around me. But surrender no longer meant giving in, it meant finding a way to do your best in the chaos of uncertainty. Covid made all worst-case scenarios a reality and I flipped from being in flow to being a survivor. Swim or die! The challenges—from financial disruption to mental instability and emotional turmoil—were a constant battle and the whole world felt like it was crumbling around me. Many business owners and sole traders were going through the same emotions, and the idea that you could lose everything you worked for in a split second was now a reality for many.

The only way out of despair was to change radically and build back up on stronger foundations. Realising that I didn't know much about money management and abundance was very confronting but it was, however, an opportunity to learn. My good friend and mentor told me to face my problems head-on so I started to study successful entrepreneurs and those who were constantly winning in various aspects of life while also inspiring others to become better versions of themselves. People like Grant Cardone, Jordan Peterson, Jack Bush, and Vandana Shiva became my inspirations as I sought hope through survival stories and tutorials on YouTube. Those lessons opened my mind to new possibilities.

Feeding my brain with valuable insights instead of crippling worries was empowering and I became intrigued by how some could create fulfilling lives through adversity. They were self-actualised: "Self-actualisation alone drives us to realise our true potential and achieve our 'ideal self'," Maslow's *Hierarchy of Needs*.

Abundance is an interesting word. It's not wealth alone—it's wealth, health, and spirit. Wealth is the ability to manifest everything you imagine in the material world. Health is about having a sharp mind, an optimum body, and a radiant spirit. In a state of abundance, one finds solace and joy in everything one does. How hard can this be? As a born strategist, I chose a pragmatic approach in my quest for abundance. I looked at the three areas of my lifestyle, my business, and myself. If I could tackle everything that was not working in each of those three areas, I would find abundance. This was my strategy. I couldn't define exactly what abundance was just yet; the only way I could do this was to work through an elimination process. Whatever didn't align with my gut feeling had to go. No more denial. No more excuses. It was time to face my lapses head-on.

FINDING PURPOSE DEMANDS COURAGE

Through my past interaction with the business world, I knew I didn't want to help the big corporations any more so I set my sights on the small business community. The little guys with great ideas, big hearts, and relentless passions. The people who tried hard but lacked the right business strategies, tactics, and processes to run more efficient businesses. Most small business owners I spoke to never had the chance to hire corporate executives. They operated from a survival mode whereas we, the executives, only operated from a domination mode.

Over coffee, I began to experience some mind-blowing discussions on various business problems that seemed unsurmountable to them, yet easy to fix for me. Those robust discussions pushed them to think bigger than they could imagine. Soon, I realised that big thinking, big ideas, and audacious goals motivated those entrepreneurs to take bigger actions. They needed someone like me to show them the way and hold them accountable. Using some of my marketing strategies, they could identify their "Mafia" offer, most profitable products, and lower-hanging fruits in one meeting. The corporate world taught me to seek profit ruthlessly. If there is no profit, there is no business. We executives do not get emotional easily, we are built to execute a plan by executing redundant products and people fast. Whatever makes the boat go faster, right? The qualities I was most ashamed of proved to be the very skills the small business community lacked. If I could use those skills to help the "underdogs," this would be my redemption.

The purpose of my business became clear: to make the world a better place, one business at a time. As soon as my purpose was verbalised, my agency was actualised. *Brand Guru Agency* was born just like that, in one weekend, my website was up by Monday, and the values were set to keep me on the right path. These were derived from my mindset hero, Kevin Roberts: "Act fast. Fail Fast. Fix fast." Without quick action, you miss great opportunities, and you overthink. Time is indeed business money. Brené Brown, *Dare to Lead*, "Leading the way takes courage and being a leader requires sacrifices." Stephen Covey, *Habit 4 Think Win-Win*, "Every transaction is a partnership; no partnership lasts unless both parties get their fair share."

Soon after, fate realigned the stars and I met Luisana, a CRM guru who became my first team member when my workload doubled in a few months. After a few months, I realised that I needed a very strong IT and Digital Strategist partner for us to be able to service larger clients. Then I met Lance when I just happened to sit next to him at a breakfast event. Very quickly there were five of us as Nat, my good friend and PR specialist, reconnected after fifteen years and I was introduced to Graz, a multimedia expert who completed our team. In less than six months, we became a multi-dimensional team of Gurus in the five key aspects of Marketing: Strategy, Customer Relations, Public Relations, Digital, and Multimedia. There was no other agency like ours on the market, a one-stop shop where you could outsource all of your marketing needs in a consistent yet flexible manner. Small business owners loved it as they felt empowered through our collaborative approach, and our business kept doubling in size every year.

IS THIS ABUNDANCE?

As the agency grew bigger, not only was the team aligned with the values, but we soon realised that the clients who stayed effortlessly and loved us dearly shared the same values and purpose. I learnt that I didn't have to compromise my values for work. This put us in a position to vet our clients; if the business and its products were not positively impacting the world, they were not a match for our agency. If the business did not contribute to the local community, then no. We did not want to be part of the "greed economy," and the more clear we became about this, the better-quality clients we attracted. They were not even clients anymore; they became friends in helping us build our vision of having more businesses with integrity in the world, businesses that valued people, quality products, healthy profits, and community growth.

As our journey evolved, we brought trust back into the label "marketing agency." Helping business owners clarify their "why, what and how" helped them plan better for their business growth and set them on a firm path of abundance. We helped a handcrafted wooden toy artisan from the farmer's market niche into educational toys and furniture. We helped a plant-based chocolate manufacturer scale on his journey to heal the world with chocolates. We helped a corporate law firm fighting to keep small businesses in the game of business. And we helped an ambitious NDIS Practitioner to build more inclusive smart cities in Africa. The agency became global. This is exactly the vision I had in mind, to help visionary entrepreneurs change the world.

But the business was just one of the three areas of my life. So to live in true abundance, I had to make changes in my lifestyle as well as in myself. I turned my attention to my mindset. *How was I holding myself and my family back? Where was I thinking too scarce?* The idea of being in your truth started to haunt me. Truth, as Dr. Peterson explains, is the only way you can manifest who you are. The truth sets you free but destroys everything that is not aligned with your truth. To avoid living a lie, I had to re-evaluate everything I say, everything I do, and everyone I associate myself with. Little did I know that to face my truth, I had to face my own lies.

Simple things such as dressing up became a question of truth. *Is this garment made in a sweatshop? Is the food processed? Is it organic?* Inspired by Vandana Shiva's work, I grew vegetables in the backyard. Living in truth was harder than I thought but I was determined to stay on the right path. I could only do it one step, habit, and reflective moment at a time. It was a lot of work to clean up my act in every little aspect of my life. I was facing the dilemma of being immersed in a consumerism culture head-on; I can't deny that I love shopping. I remembered my discussion with Bandana Tewari in Bali when she told me she only buys things she is madly in love with. "Fashion is like wearing a piece of art," she said. This made a lot of sense now and was a way to reconcile my love of shopping with my heart. *Why don't we buy things that we will love forever? Why don't we cherish objects like we used to in the past?* After the process of shedding the old self, belongings, and some relationships, living an abundant life was about finding joy in every moment. Through awareness, you can stop recurring patterns; as Joe Dispenza says beautifully, "If we cannot think greater than how we feel, we cannot change." I was determined to change, so I started visualising myself as my better and future self.

Walking the path of truth was a confronting one, to say the least, and I keep experiencing my fragmented self as I realise how much more I have to grow. Facing my flaws was my road to redemption. I was not blaming my relatives, my situation, or the economy anymore—I was taking full responsibility for my life. Gathering the courage to face my shortcomings revealed untapped potential. I decided to believe in the truth by forgiving myself first and then forgiving others.

Trust is something I had to grapple with in the discovery of forgiveness. Trust is finding the courage to believe in people. Knowing I can find the courage to trust in the future no matter what; in me alone is the ability to overcome adversity, betrayals, and even sickness. The old saying that what doesn't kill you makes you stronger became my truth, and the only way I could face the future is through resilience. There is neither a perfect nor an ideal future. There are not even expectations to be had. There is hope, courage, and determination to stay in the abundance vibration aligned with my Big Hairy Audacious Goal to make this world a better place. And if I faltered, I learnt to be compassionate with myself by focusing on what I did better this time compared to the previous time. My focus is to be a better person, wife, mother, and leader. Not the best, just better than yesterday. As I hold myself accountable, I keep raising the standard of my life. I love myself more and gain more respect for my character. At the same time, my commitment to a better life inspired my close family and friends to do the same. Although I cannot change anyone, I can still lead the way.

ABOUT THE AUTHOR

DEENA SYED

Deena Syed is a seasoned Brand Strategist with twenty years of experience working with iconic Australian brands, helping them increase their market share and develop sustainable business growth strategies.

She has the unique ability to bring business strategy to fruition with hands-on creative executions. Her talent and passion combined with a deep understanding of neuro-marketing makes her a great asset to any business looking for emotional connections with its target market.

In 2020, Deena founded Brand Guru Agency, as she saw a gap in the market for a full-service outsourced marketing one-stop shop. She now helps smaller businesses dream big and take bigger actions to make positive changes in the world. Brand Guru offers marketing strategy, branding expertise, and advertising services to over one hundred small-to-medium-sized businesses across Australia, and is growing fast as a niche, integrated full-service agency.

CONNECT WITH DEENA HERE:

Website: www.brandguruagency.com

Free Gift: https://brandguruagency.com/bhag

Contact: https://brandguruagency.com/contact-us

JEN PORTEOUS

WOMEN OF THE KINGDOM

DESCENDING INTO THE FEMININE HEART TO RESTORE OUR RELATIONSHIP WITH THE MASCULINE

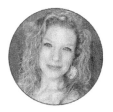

WHO IS A WOMAN OF THE KINGDOM?

*S*he is the expression of God's heart. His vessel. Stewarding all that he has blessed her with. She embodies the knowing that she is a daughter to the King, and she has a higher calling than ownership: her stewardship. Her wisdom and feminine truth is the balm for all those she is meant to reach. She moves in truth as a way of being.

The Feminine Heart, in all its raw, beautiful truth, is the source for inspiration and emanation of love. She was born this way. This is her original, organic design.

To see our hearts, our feelings, our needs, our desires, and share them with open vulnerability is the deepest safety we can experience. It sends the message that we are worthy and we are seen. "I can share myself in truth because I am valid. My feelings are valid, my needs are valid, my desires are valid. I am worthy simply because I am. Because I exist. I am a daughter of God."

Godly femininity is a state of being within her true identity. When we are anchored in truth, how our feminine is expressed to the world will look different than the woman standing beside us, but our soft, penetrable hearts, open to receive, will be felt even before we enter a room or open our mouths. There is nothing to be lost other than armor we have been hiding behind and building for our entire lives. We only remember our true self.

There is no loss of your competency. Letting go of your perceptions of what it means to be feminine enables you to open yourself up to expressing your unique expression of femininity to the world. When men say they want an independent woman, they don't mean a woman independent of needing him, but a woman who is independent of who she is in her own agency. She is free from the armor of judgment, shame, and unworthiness.

She can still run a business, change a tire, ride a motorcycle, be cheeky and sassy, shoot a gun, or none of those things. What brings her joy and excitement while honoring her heart at all times, is the truth of the feminine. But our judgment is what keeps us from experiencing our deepest freedom. The feminine has had so many stereotypes attached to it over the years. That we must look, dress, speak, and act in a certain way. In our minds we have also created a version of the feminine that we reject and don't identify with, so we tell ourselves we are not "feminine" or "feminine enough." And so we betray ourselves, over and over.

I know this. I know it well, because I did it. I betrayed myself over and over every single time I said "yes" when I needed to say "no." When I changed how I expressed myself to men because I was told they didn't like it and couldn't handle it. When I stopped doing certain things because "other people won't like it." When I allowed people to keep hurting me and I never said anything. When I thought if I just loved them more, then that would inspire them to love me better. All it did was deplete me. Erode my self-worth. And leave me feeling ashamed, alone, and unfulfilled.

The invitation in the submission to your heart is to release yourself from all of that above. To deepen back into the deep feeling, expressive vessel that you are as a woman of God and the Kingdom. Our self-love is determined by nothing other than our willingness to see ourselves as whole, and the intention and expression to honor it radically, the way God designed us.

Since we were children, in most cases we have been brainwashed into proving that we are perfect, and that if we are not perfect, we are not enough or loveable. The proving of our worth through controlling, hustling, leading, pushing. We have been slowly conditioned to operate from a fragmented, immature feminine. The feminine heart yearns to be seen, held, kept, and contained. We were created for expression. And yet somewhere when we were small, we learned to manipulate because we knew no other way to get our needs met if we were not perfect.

BUT WHAT IS MANIPULATION?

It always comes with a subtle tone of malicious intent attached to it. Reframing how we view manipulation is how we learn to refine ourselves to move away from it, to learn the cues of our body when we are in it. They are usually obvious but we have learned to ignore them. All it was, originally, was a way to get our needs met.

Any time we do or say *anything* with the intention of outcome, it is manipulation. Outcomes can look like many things. Things we may not consider to be outcomes at first. When we perform, or hide certain parts of ourselves, we are manipulating. We are attempting to control how the other person perceives us—to be liked, desired, accepted, wanted. The root of this is fear of rejection. "If I show all of me and they don't like me, I am rejected." And it's *painful*. The consequence is that we know that we are never really being seen completely and loved for the truth of who we are. If you are not sharing from truth, you cannot be seen entirely, and you cannot trust that whatever outcome occurs is happening because it was meant to because you are seen, or because you manipulated. If there is even an outcome at all.

This will affirm a belief of feeling unworthy, unseen, insignificant, and not enough. The cycle of people-pleasing, and perfectionism repeats, exhausting the body and heart.

I used to say, "I miss you" or, "I love you," not because perhaps I didn't miss or love them, but because there was a deep yearning in me that wanted to hear it. I was saying it to have it said back. I had a need to feel loved and had no idea how to say, " I feel lonely and need love and attention right now." The manipulation was saying it first in the hope my sentiments would be returned. Those words often were, but deep down I never knew if it was true or not because it was entirely possible that they were saying it just because I did. It wasn't malicious. I simply had no idea how to access and express the truth of my need. I didn't even know that's what I did need.

THERE IS A LOT OF MESSAGING OUT THERE ABOUT THE TRUTH

And "one truth" and "our truth" and the endless searching many people have for the truth. What is it? Where is it?

The vibration of truth is universally recognized, consciously or subconsciously, regardless of faith or beliefs, because it carries its own frequency and is higher and above all else. It can be felt before words are said. The vibration of truth resonates in our bodies and in the bodies of others. It is *felt*. The vibration of truth is completely clean of manipulation. This is why the feminine is so powerful when she moves herself into the natural expression of her heart. She vibrates in truth. The sword of truth, in all its purity.

If there is even a hint of manipulation, it will feel distorted in her body. And that distortion will be felt by whoever she is sharing herself with, even if it's just herself.

It's in this pure frequency only, that we feel seen. Either by our own self, or by others. We cannot be fully seen, or felt, if there is any distortion attached to our expression. This is the deepest and hardest part: to clear ourselves of manipulation. Only when we express the truth do we truly respect ourselves and each other.

Over the course of our lives, we move upward into our heads. Thinking our way through experiences instead of feeling our way through them and *being* in them. We lose the language of our bodies that we were born with. Numbed, ignored, suppressed and shamed. We feel shame for wanting anything. Needing anything. We feel shame for feeling sad, lonely, imperfect, and for needing a man.

Our society constantly sends a message that heavier emotions make you *less*. If you are not perfect all the time, you are less. Men don't want a woman who is difficult, who is anything other than independent, successful, happy, and sexual. But women don't *need* a man either. A woman who needs a man is also less. We become so detached, we often don't even know what our needs are. We don't even know our own truth.

I never was able to see how a man provided safety that I couldn't provide for myself.

I usually made more money. I could drive. Run my house. Change a tire. Manage my life. Take care of my children. I could cook, clean, and run things like clockwork.

AND HERE COMES THE LIE

If we can do it, we don't need a man. They are a perk, a bonus, a want. Not a need.

But, I have sons. And this weighed heavily on my heart. What message was I sending to my boys about their significance in life, marriage, and love? *That they were not of value because they were going to grow up to be men.* I can't even begin to describe the gut-wrenching pain this caused me. My two amazing sons—not valuable? Disposable? That women could take them or leave them? I felt sick to my stomach over that thought.

Layered with my own deep lack of fulfillment, despite doing everything "right," I was still longing for that safety, and I wasn't even convinced that it existed or was possible for me.

Could a man really meet me at my depth? I held a belief that maybe it just wasn't in the cards for me. And yet, I couldn't let it go. My heart would not let it go.

To my sons, the consequences of my belief system were too great. I had to be willing to put down my shields. And I didn't even know what most of them were. But I did know that I was in my mid-thirties and none of the "right" things I was doing felt good, or were bringing me any closer to what was in my heart. The only feeling I could access was exhaustion. Releasing all the judgment, manipulation, shame, and old beliefs was the only way; and I had carried them for as long as I could remember. It was a very deep and long journey of reconnecting to my heart and body, and restoring my identity. The restoration of my femininity, my daughterhood, and truth. A journey so deep that I didn't realize how heavy it had all been until I wasn't carrying it anymore and felt the clarity of what I had been numb to for almost my entire adult life. The subconscious shame had consumed me.

MY REALIZATIONS

1. I had no idea that my deepest relief was in the deliverance from the subconscious agony of shame.

2. Shame was the heaviest weight I had ever carried without knowing how much I was holding.

3. I felt shame for needing God, a man, money, protection, and safety.

I discovered that men are a physical representation of the masculine energy of God. Therefore, I cannot judge men without also judging all masculine energy, and God. All that provides for me, protects me, and is devotional to me. I cannot judge one without judging all. I was called to truly see men in a new light.

ALL OF THIS IS A REFLECTION OF OUR RELATIONSHIP WITH GOD

When we can learn to rest in faith, rest in the love that we receive from *Him*, but before a man steps in to fulfill the role as your masculine partner in life, we must cultivate this relationship with God. For most, this will be the most difficult part. To put the "doing" down. To do less. To surrender to God's pace and plan. To be led by his timing. This is the ultimate surrender. To acknowledge our tension, breathe into the edges that are being pressed against because we are not "making it happen." There is no force. No pushing. We are truly led women. Our modern society makes it easier than ever to do everything ourselves. To obtain instant gratification with a single text, social media, random encounters, dating apps, and "boss babe-ing."

TO BE A GOD-LED WOMAN IS NO EASY FEAT IN TODAY'S WORLD

A world that encourages us to self-abandon at every corner, that sends the message that we need to do it all to feel safe, that detaches us from the true expression of our heart's needs, feelings, and desires. Being a God-led woman is the complete destruction of everything we have ever told ourselves, and had others tell us we are. And to be seen, the way God sees us. To see ourselves, the way God made us. To love ourselves the way God loves us. This is our faith.

Our faith that, as we shed each layer and expose the raw vulnerability of who we are to the world, we will be protected, even without all the armor that the world has told us we need to be safe. The depths in which we are willing to be obliterated are the same depths in which we are able to receive love. To Honor the love that we have always been worthy of. It's how we say "Yes" to receiving all the love that is included in being the daughter of a king. It's how we say "Yes, I see myself the way you see me."

To shed false identity until there is nothing left but the truth. The truth of our raw, vulnerable hearts. So exposed that it feels dangerous and yet contained. Because we are protected. The masculine can feel our vulnerability and rises to protect us fiercely. The irony being that we cannot receive protection without the faith that when we are stripped of our armor, we will still be protected. And that we do not need to self-protect. We must be willing to be vulnerable first, to move in faith and trust first, and then the masculine will rise. This is the inspiration. Anything done before we are moving in faith is done from manipulation. This is most often seen in our relationship with men.

MEN WHO FEEL MANIPULATED

Men feel manipulated too; even subtly they will often have no desire to meet women's needs, wants, or desires. And life, money, and business respond the same way. And if they do, it's from the space of obligation and people-pleasing. The minute we manipulate anyone, we disrespect ourselves and them at the same time.

Manipulation is disrespectful to their freedom to respond from their authenticity. Even if she gets what she wants, it will not be received with trust at a core level because she didn't share the vulnerable truth. It will always be a transaction when we function from the energy of manipulation. Something, deep down will never feel completely fulfilled because our subconscious knows we weren't in our authenticity and integrity.

In his humanness, he is going to fail. He's going to make mistakes. He's going to hit speed bumps and difficult situations. He will not always know what to do right away. And this is where we anchor into our love and our devotion. And most importantly, our feminine grace.

Our expectations that men need to be perfect for us to give them our love, time, compassion, devotion, and bodies is merely a reflection of how we treat ourselves. That we need to be perfect and performative before we see ourselves with love, devotion, and grace. And it can absolutely rock you. You will feel the urge burning inside you to fix, solve, advise, and mother him. It's in these moments, that we are invited to see the king in our men. To anchor into our trust and faith that he can and will figure it out. Even when it's hard. Even when we are suffering with him. We suffer because the person we love is suffering. Our ability to hold this sensation and anchor in our faith in him even when we feel the chaos inside of us is the expression of our love and devotion. We respect him because we honor the man we know and believe he is.

DEVELOPING TRUST AND FAITH IN OUR MEN

The expression of this trust and faith to our men, when centered from our devotion and truth, is where we uphold our values as Kingdom women. His rising into his fullest potential is *his* choice. The call of the masculine to rise is always his own journey, and own initiation. It cannot be forced or coerced. Men know when they are being manipulated. Even if this is not a conscious knowing; their subconscious does.

Our men are human. It is not their responsibility to meet our every whim, desire, and demand. Our entire society has moved into a paradigm that a man who does not do these things is not a man who deserves you. Sorry, Sister. This couldn't be further from the truth.

There is so much more to expand on in this journey we take as women, into the remembrance of our original femininity. This is explored in depth and clarified in my mentorship programs, website, and social media pages.

If you have resonated with my journey from the manipulating people-pleasing, hustling, woman into that reclamation of a woman of the Kingdom, I invite you to join me on this journey so that, together, we can change the dynamics and dysfunctionality in relationships, as we each step into the soft, restful version of who we truly are.

There is a woman of the Kingdom within you, waiting to be remembered. Let me be your steward, let me be your guide.

ABOUT THE AUTHOR

JEN PORTEOUS

After eighteen years of hustle, grind, boss-babe culture, Jen realized that she had become numb, detached, anxious, overworked, and stressed. She couldn't sleep at night. Her neutrality had come to mean that she was "happy."

Without a plan, she walked away from her career field to figure out what it meant to feel and be a feminine woman of God in a world that demanded she be anything but that.

Jen now helps women to gain a deeper understanding and fully embody their femininity as women of the Kingdom. Restoring daughterhood, where they no longer disrupt their health, relationships, and families in the process, and to energetically shift from that hustle anxiety-filled culture to naturally softer, feminine truth and authenticity. Stewarding their own unique design and purpose.

Three years on, she's not that same person. Jen sleeps at night, her heart is at rest, she feels the full range of her feminine, and lets her spirit and faith guide her to being the woman she is so much more comfortable and at peace with as a woman of the Kingdom.

CONNECT WITH JEN HERE:

Website: https://kingdom-femininity.com

Instagram: https://www.instagram.com/kingdom_femininity_restoration/

RASHEEDAH BILAL

RADICAL ACCOUNTABILITY

A PERSONAL LIBERATION MANIFESTO

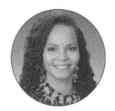

*E*ssential to self-empowerment is acknowledging your part in your own suffering. This may not be easy to hear. Stay with me.

Acknowledging the choices you have made and understanding their consequences is the first step towards transformation. *But if it were so straightforward, then why are so many of us still struggling?* This chapter explores these challenges and provides possible answers to inspire you to embrace your own power in a new way.

PART I–STASIS

"And that's why we're not going with this vendor." Jared looked pretty pleased with his presentation, "And now..."

"Actually," Rachel's smooth, low voice sliced through the air like a sword, "I would like to go back a few slides." Jared lifted his head, surprised by her sudden demand. "Uh, sure." He clicked back on the slideshow, the projector flickering as it adjusted to the previous slide.

Rachel leaned forward, her eyes fixed on the screen. A pen twirled through her long, slender fingers, her expression thoughtful as Jared clicked back through his presentation. "There. Stop on this slide. Now, maybe only I missed your explanation," she said slowly, her voice low and sultry, as she glanced up at Jared, leaned back in her seat and confidently scanned the whole boardroom, "but humor me and walk us through the details of this chart. Talk to me like I'm two."

Lila was seated in the back corner of the room; to her, Rachel's presence was undeniable. Her voice filled the air with a confidence that could not be overlooked and her dark eyes pierced every soul in the room. Rachel seemed to know exactly what she was talking about and everyone held their breath, waiting for her next clever observation.

Lila looked on in admiration as Rachel broke down Jared's presentation. She spoke with such conviction and command that the room seemed to fill with her words, captivating every ear. Both impressed and intimidated, Lila knew her own abilities couldn't compare to Rachel's eloquence and expertise.

Jared seemed to sense this as he quickly replied to each of Rachel's questions, taking her through every detail on the chart with an almost dogged determination. Despite his obvious admiration for Rachel, Lila could tell that he was trying his best not to get too flustered in front of her.

"Damn. What a bad bitch!" Lila was in awe of Rachel, the most junior board member, dominating the conversation. She exuded control and self-assurance with her sharp gaze and calm demeanor. Watching her, Lila admired her brilliance and confidence, feeling that she'd make a great friend. When Rachel made her motion to go with a certain vendor, everyone exhaled as Lila smiled, completely understanding why they were drawn to Rachel's conviction and audacity.

Feeling bold, Lila approached Rachel, took a deep breath and cleared her throat. "Hey, Rachel," she said confidently, although her voice trembled slightly, "Man, I heard rumors about your briefing style. It's quite something to watch in person. I've been here for fifteen years and I still doubt myself when I'm briefing. I don't know how you don't get tired of constantly being questioned by men. I see them get frustrated with me when I simply ask a question; those slight snickers as though I'm the only one who doesn't know something we should all know." Lila leaned in, let out a frustrated sigh, and with an almost desperate tone asked, "Seriously though. How do you do it? Call men on their bullshit but somehow seem to be respected all at once?"

Rachel looked up with a small smile on her lips. She couldn't help but notice that Lila had worked herself up and quickly assessed that this conversation was going to take up the rest of her afternoon. Years of experience also made her very attuned to recognize a bid for attention when it was presented to her. "Thank you, Lila. That means a lot coming from someone with your experience." Rachel's gaze was warm and kind, making Lila feel instantly at ease. Rachel started to walk towards the exit and indicated for Lila to join her.

"You know, Lila, there is no reason to doubt yourself; you have a lot of knowledge and experience that I could learn from."

Lila felt herself blush at Rachel's words. "Thank you," she replied, feeling grateful for Rachel's encouragement. "I was wondering if, maybe, we could grab lunch sometime? I'd love to pick your brain about your approach to the briefing and see if there's anything I can learn from you."

Rachel's smile widened, "Funny you should mention lunch, I was going to ask you the same thing." Rachel glanced down at her watch, "How about now? I'm a huge fan of the little Thai bistro two blocks down. If your afternoon is open we can meet in the front lobby in fifteen minutes and walk together?"

Lila perked up with excitement. "That sounds great, Rachel. Let me clear my afternoon and I'll meet you downstairs."

Rachel canceled her afternoon meetings with a swift text to her assistant.

Sitting at her desk, Rachel thought back to the days of her early twenties when, despite her sharp wit and engaging personality, she had been crippled with the burden of insecurity and stayed in survival mode. She ran her fingers across her empowerment tattoo on her left wrist, "I am, therefore I am." A reminder of the intense relationship fifteen years ago that helped change her course. Now, Rachel was exactly where she should be—oozing knowledge and empowering those around her.

Feeling anticipation, she strode confidently towards the lobby. This was a chance to teach and learn. She couldn't help but wonder what the future held for them and their organization.

PART II–TRIUMPH

"Starving!" Rachel exclaimed, grinning. She usually fasted intermittently but was too busy the day before to eat. A spin class had sapped her last ounce of energy. Opening the door wide, she stepped aside and gestured for Lila to enter.

They sat at a small table by the window and studied the menu. After ordering drinks, Lila looked at Rachel with awe and envy, wondering how she remained so poised in meetings. Rachel leaned back, took a sip of lemon water and said calmly, "Would you believe I once was homeless?"

Lila was stunned by the revelation. She had never expected to hear something like that, and she could tell from the serious expression on Rachel's face that she wasn't joking.

Rachel recounted, "After college, I went to Boston in search of a job and to kickstart my career. Things didn't go as I'd hoped and I ended up living out of my car for a while. In this period, I met an incredible man with whom I had a very intense but short relationship. At the time, when it ended, I was heartbroken, but in hindsight I feel that he was my guardian angel sent to grant me the knowledge I was missing."

Rachel paused, her eyes steadily meeting Lila's with just a hint of sadness. "But even that wasn't the worst of it," she said softly. She continued in a more forceful tone, "A few weeks later I attended a job fair with a friend and thought I had found my solution—joining the military. Little did I know I was signing up for a real nightmare."

Rachel took another sip of her lemon water as she looked around to catch the server's eye and waved him over. "I say nightmare, but I served for fifteen years." Rachel had a twinkle in her eye as she looked across at Lila, "You see, this was also the chapter in my life where I finally used—

correction, found myself with no other option but to use—the wisdom my guardian angel had left me with so, so many years ago."

Lila was mesmerized by Rachel's words and the person who was emerging in front of her. She had never thought that someone as powerful as Rachel could possibly have gone through so much in the past. "What did he teach you, Rachel?" she asked eagerly, leaning forward.

Rachel smiled warmly at Lila. "More on that a little later," she said with a wave of her hand, gesturing to the menu in front of them. "Let's order some food."

As they ate, Rachel gave Lila a glimpse of her past, from her childhood to college days to the year she spent homeless, and finally her time in the military. Lila was completely captivated by her story, laughing at her humorous anecdotes while feeling even more admiration for someone who had gone through so much and could tell her story with such eloquence.

"Thanks," she said as she gave the last plate to the waiter, "Can you bring us a bottle of chardonnay and two glasses?" She winked at Lila, "I thought you'd like something to give you some confidence." "What do you mean? I'm not scared!" Lila laughed nervously. Rachel reached out and held both of Lila's hands in her own. "We can have a chat about methods on building self-esteem, or how to make an impression, or I can give you an exercise that I use with other women that shows my perspective on being a female in a male-dominated industry. But I have to ask, are you looking for a sounding board or simply an echo chamber?"

Lila took a moment to consider Rachel's question. "I want both," she finally said, "I want someone who can listen to me and offer their perspective, but I also want someone who can challenge me and help me grow."

Rachel nodded thoughtfully. "I can do that," she said, pouring the wine and handing Lila a glass. "Let's do this then."

Lila leaned in, eager to hear what Rachel had to say.

"I want you to take a moment," Rachel said, "and think back to a situation that made you feel small or insignificant—maybe it was a meeting where you didn't feel heard, or a project where you felt like your ideas were dismissed. Whatever it is, I want you to recall it in detail." Rachel took a sip of wine, "When you have it, tell me how you remember it happening."

"I've been in the same position for almost five years and I don't think I'm going anywhere anytime soon. I feel like my thoughts are always overlooked during meetings and my boss appears to favor the male members of the team over me. My capabilities are just as good as theirs, but it doesn't seem like I'm given the same chances. A couple of months ago, I proposed an idea to my superior but he didn't even consider it; he simply disregarded it and moved on to another subject. That left me feeling like my opinions didn't matter. Then last week they promoted Mike—he only has two years under his belt with us and I can tell it's because he and the boss golf together." Lila was getting more and more worked up. "It feels like I work twice as hard as everyone else here," she said.

"Let's take last week when we had a meeting with a client for the latest project." Rachel frowned as she fixed her eyes on Lila. "So, what happened there?"

"I had been working on the proposal for ages," Lila said, a hint of dejection in her voice. "But when I presented it to my boss, he completely ignored me. The moment Mike mentioned his own haphazard plan though, my supervisor went absolutely wild with enthusiasm. It was totally infuriating. When I tried to speak my mind again, someone even rolled their eyes and said that this kind of thing should be left to 'the grown-ups'."

Lila discussed her struggles further; she wasn't scared, more like drained from working in a male-dominated field. "It's really tiring," she said. "I feel like I'm constantly walking this tightrope between being compassionate but disregarded, or being assertive but then getting criticized in my performance reviews for being too pushy. I just feel like I have to walk a thin line being compassionate, yet dismissed, or being assertive and being told in my evaluations that I'm abrasive."

"Why can't they just accept me?" she said with frustration, "I had to go to HR a few years back and now it feels like I'm almost punished for standing up to them when they're unfair. But I have every right to make sure they understand their wrongdoings." She stared at Rachel as if she wanted her approval.

Rachel refilled their glasses and took a sip of her own. Her gaze rested on Lila's as she spoke, saying, "I get why you feel like the system is working against you; it's hard to struggle all the time."

Lila nervously chuckled and swirled her wine around in the glass. "So, can you tell me your secret? How can I be like you, brave and never discouraged?"

"Stop allowing yourself to be a victim," Rachel replied.

Lila was taken aback by the words and her tone. "Excuse me?"

Rachel's gaze was gentle. "From what I've seen, women want a seat at the table while needing to hear others affirm their right to be there. They want autonomy but also dependency." She paused for a moment, "We yearn for the strength of self-reliance, yet cling to the allure of unattained innocence—a dichotomy begging to be shattered."

Lila frowned, confused by Rachel's words and feeling a little defensive. "I don't understand what you mean by that," she said.

Rachel leaned forward, her eyes bright with intensity. "Here's the thing, Lila—you can't have both. You can't expect to be treated as an equal and also be coddled. You have to be strong enough to take your seat at the table, to assert yourself, to fight for what you believe in. You can't wait for someone else to give you permission to be there."

"Are you saying discrimination doesn't happen? Can you honestly say that Mark, Peter and the team aren't given preferential treatment because they're men?" Lila asked as she drained the last of her wine glass. "I think we need another bottle," she said, gesturing for the server.

"Well you're treating, so why not?" Rachel chuckled as she winked at Lila, causing her to loosen up a bit. "I want you to hear this message clearly. What other people do will always be *their* business. Your job is to *not* be naive about what is *their* business and own every single one of *your* choices."

"I don't follow," Lila poured them both a glass, "What does that have to do with how they treat me at work? None of that is my fault."

"It's called radical accountability. You don't get to play innocent or act naive when you decide to be the author of your own story." Rachel paused for a moment to let her words sink in before continuing. "Yes, discrimination exists and it's not fair. But at some point, you have to stop focusing on what others are doing and start taking control of your own actions."

Lila's brow furrowed as she tried to digest Rachel's words. "But how do I do that? How do I take control?"

Rachel grinned. "By using the 'I' narrative. Where you're only allowed to recount stories from the perspective of your actions and choices." Rachel's voice was smooth yet powerful, "And fall out of love with the notion that someone else is coming to secure *your* seat at any table at which you want to have a seat."

Lila didn't seem to believe her. "How is this supposed to help me?"

"Let's put that into practice for the second half of the exercise, okay?" Lila nodded as Rachel continued, "I want you to retell the story about the project with the new clients. But this time, you can only retell it using the 'I' narrative."

Lila took a deep breath and closed her eyes for a moment, gathering her thoughts. When she opened them again, she began to speak, "I had been honing the proposal for weeks, and I was proud of it," she said, her voice growing stronger. "But when I presented it to my team, my boss seemed uninterested. He wasn't even listening to what I had to say. I felt angry and frustrated, but rather than speaking up and asking him to pay attention, I just stayed quiet and let him talk over me."

Rachel smiled as she interrupted. "When you told the story the first time, you focused on how everyone else acted. Now, try to focus only on what you did in this situation. You interpreted your boss's silence as disregard and used it as an excuse to stay quiet."

"Well, he *did* disregard me," Lila said a little defensively.

"Innocence over agency. And *you* chose to give it weight and affect your next choices in a way that allows you today to be a victim." Rachel shot back, "And what happened next?"

"That's when Mike spoke up," Lila said, a slight edge to her voice. "He presented his own plan, which was much less thought out than mine, but my boss seemed to love it. And when I tried to speak up again, someone rolled their eyes and told me to let the grown-ups handle it."

"Let's fix your story," Rachel said, taking a sip from her glass." Use only 'I' sentences."

Lila inhaled deeply before continuing. "Mike made his proposal and I felt overwhelmed when my boss agreed with the most mediocre, dull, ill-conceived idea."

"Ah, there it is—the fire in your eyes!" Rachel smiled encouragingly. "Good job! Keep going."

"I wanted to speak up and tell them that my proposal was much better, but I hesitated. I was worried about coming across as too pushy or aggressive. So instead, I just sat there and seethed silently."

Rachel nodded encouragingly. "And what did that accomplish?"

Lila let out a small sigh, her voice trailing off, "I felt so insignificant and helpless. I should've told my boss that I expect the same respect from him as he gives to others, and also asked him to tell people not to treat me in such a rude way."

"You could do that," Rachel said, "But why not be a badass instead?" At this, she let out a low chuckle.

"Sure, you could demand fairness from your boss, draw attention to the mistreatment you're experiencing, or even take it to HR or another relevant department. But if you want my advice, it's learning the art of being your own hero. Stand up for yourself, be your own champion, use humor when appropriate."

She continued. "For example, if someone made a comment like 'leave it to the grown-ups' when they rolled their eyes at you? A smart response might be 'Well that disqualifies you because your work is similar to my twelve-year-old son's.'"

Lila laughed at the response, feeling a newfound confidence growing within her. "I like that," she said. "It's funny, but also assertive."

Rachel grinned. "Exactly. And it shows that you won't stand for being dismissed or belittled. You can still be professional and confident while standing up for yourself and asserting your worth."

Lila nodded in agreement. "I think I get it now. I need to focus on what I can control and use my voice to assert myself, rather than waiting for someone else to do it for me."

"Exactly," Rachel said, raising her glass in a toast. "Here's to being our own heroes," she said with a smile," and never waiting for someone else to secure our seat at the table."

Like Rachel in this story, I am devoted to helping people find their voice, own their narratives, and become their own heroes. It's amazing to see people change from feeling powerless and hopeless to being able to stand up for themselves without question. Not only in the office setting but in all aspects of life, I educate the use of the "I" narrative to bring consciousness to our decisions and recognize how much influence we have over our situations and eventual outcomes. It is my hope that you cultivate a deep awareness of how powerful you really are. As you move forward, embrace the liberation that brings forth a more empowered and fulfilled life.

ABOUT THE AUTHOR

RASHEEDAH BILAL

Rasheedah Bilal is regarded as an exceptional leader in the US Army who has garnered personal and professional admiration from those around her. Growing up in Saudi Arabia, Rasheedah is no stranger to picking her own path in the face of adversity. This mindset served her throughout her journey earning a reputation as a standout female role model.

"Who else shows up to a driving test and expects to pass without having driven a car before?" and "A down-ass chick I would call if I wanted to take over a country," is how people describe her.

What makes her leadership style unique is its remarkable impact. Characterized by her candor, palpable grit, tenacity, and exceptional ability to mentor individuals at all levels, she serves as a dynamic influencer, who motivates individuals to empower themselves as catalysts of positive change.

Rasheedah is currently working on a leadership podcast for 2024 and in her free time, is building her own Harley Davidson motorcycle.

CONNECT WITH RASHEEDAH HERE:

For all socials and links: https://linktr.ee/rbilal

CRAIG WHITNEY

HOW TO GIVE YOURSELF A SECOND CHANCE

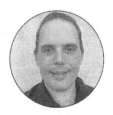

*H*ave you ever given yourself a second chance? If so, how has

that impacted your life? Are you making a difference and creating an impact in your world today?

I have found that we give ourselves a second chance by default for every challenge we face. The definition of a second chance is to get up once more and try again. How does this shape our life? Do we emulate the behaviours that we have either witnessed or experienced at earlier times in our lives? Yes, we do—by default. They are ingrained in our nervous system, build up over years of suppressed experiences, and often come out in our later years.

SOCIETY'S PRESSURE TO MAKE IT AS A MAN

Think about the pressures we live under as men. We are inherently providers. We work long hours to provide for our families. We are told to man up. Stop crying. Hit the gym. Overwhelmed by ten thousand different stereotypes of obsolete warrior archetypes of what it is to be a man. Growing up we are taught, by no fault of our fathers, that crying or

124

showing emotions is a sign of weakness. Which, publicly, it is. In the workplace men need to take a stoic stance in some professions. There's a time and space for that.

Single-parent household and your mother may have raised you by herself, or co-parented your upbringing, or maybe you had many different styles of fatherly role models in your life as you grew up? Maybe you're a man sitting there after a situation, feeling overwhelm creeping in—what do I do now? You know you have acted in a way that has consequences, so the anxiety creeps in. Or you're a man in your mid-thirties; married to a childhood sweetheart, two kids, a house and two cars, and the pressures of societal conditioning to perform as a man place you in a state of total overwhelm and confusion. In a place of not knowing where to go. Your significant other is expecting you to lead and provide, and you feel you can't give any more. Or you're a man who is so overwhelmed by personal development, like I was at the tipping point of my crisis. I bought every book, but studying, however, fed my ego, not my heart and mind.

My name is Craig Whitney. I am a *Second Chance Man*. I have been through situations where I have acted out violently. Been punished. Publicly shamed in the media. Attempted suicide. All resulted from acting on the impulse of untreated childhood trauma that came out in my early thirties. I have spent over five years rebuilding myself. Learning to give myself a second chance and do it and not try. Showing up every day and doing the inner work is a daily battle to become a new way of being amongst ten thousand different stereotypes of what our culture defines a man to be. After sitting in numerous amazing men's circles, I see that, yes, they have similarities, but some are also outdated lenses from the civil rights era, and beyond that back to our primal roots. In today's age of manhood, however, our predators have not simply become extinct, but have morphed into something else.

A MOB OF WILD DONKEYS RAISED ME

This sums up my early childhood. Growing up on a cattle farm with a father who did his best as a grazier and council worker to provide under a matriarchal family model where mum was in charge. Post-depression colonist values where the son follows the father around to learn the skills of the land, in turn as an only son, to inherit the family farm later in life.

My mother was a passionate RSPCA advocate and donkey lover. She ran her own business as a stallholder providing donkey rides to impoverished kids at local markets, fetes, shows, and festivals. They were even movie stars in *Crocodile Dundee* which was filmed at Mudgeeraba on the Gold Coast in the early 1980s before the "dozers" moved in. When mum wasn't travelling around the countryside working shows, she advocated donkey rescues and rehoming.

When it came to discipline, my parents were very much old-fashioned. Treated by a stick, belt, stockwhip or sulkie whip to, "Be good, or else!" and "Children are seen and not heard," these mantras were repeated frequently by my mother. This, alongside traditional farming practices, now viewed as cruel and barbaric: hot branding of cattle and "earmarking"—where a chunk of a cow's ear is cut out with a pocket knife in the initial castration—was intimidating. What senior stockmen do. Instead of a vet.

Often when I was naughty and acted up, I received brutal floggings from my mother. Eventually, there was one too many; the final straw broke one day: June the Second, 1995. A day after *Beef Week 1995* in Casino, I was beaten badly with a stockwhip and rubber mallet, which left bruises on me the size of dinner plates. My parents had been warned by "Child Safety" to stop these out-of-date methods but my mother, as the dominant figure in the house, didn't. Off to school I went for the last time, as I was taken by Child Safety, put into foster care, and made a ward of the state. I was one of the early cases in the New South Wales "Anti-smacking" legislation that came into effect in 1995.

From the age of nine I grew up in foster care which, while being a complete shock to the system, was an experience I will forever be grateful for. If not for this reset in my life, I may have turned out like my father. Instead, I had a loving family and foster siblings with kids coming from all walks of life who were put into foster care and, overall, the Department of Community Services system as it was called then.

On the flip side, I grew up with a family who raced greyhounds for a living and live-baited dogs. I witnessed greyhounds going missing, winning and losing money, and rabbits and chickens being mauled to death, all in the name of sport. These family traditions had an impact. My foster parents did what was necessary to provide for the family because they were, and still are, passionate carers for kids in desperate need.

Until the age of fourteen, I was a nerd at school—up until my mother finally died from an epic two-year battle with cancer. That set me off the rails. Going from a B-grade student to class rebel, I pretty much failed high school and began to experiment with marijuana. Over the next couple of years, I received many school suspensions for grass clippings, parsley, and contaminated marijuana; all in the name of going to a public school in Australia.

After leaving school at seventeen for a stint at TAFE (a local Vocational college) and a failed attempt to enter the Navy, I floated. Living on government benefits and studying part-time, my foster dad gave me a choice of either studying full-time, or moving out and getting a job. So I moved out. I got a good break, moved to Casino and worked at a couple of sawmills before being lured out to Inverell by my two best mates from high school, Mat and Matthew, who worked at a local abattoir.

On the ANZAC Day long weekend in 2005, I moved to Inverell, a small country town in western New South Wales. This is where I made my debut in the beef industry—and had my craziest life experiences! Mat, Matthew and I all drank and partied like crazy. We had girlfriends and slept with each other's girlfriends. I even slept with crazed married women, which I unknowingly paid for at the time. This time in my life centred my career in the abattoir environment and set my goals. By October 2007, my friendship with the Matts was made, and we all moved out of Inverell. Both Matt and Matthew moved back to Casino and I moved to Brisbane where I got a start at another bigger abattoir and finished learning my trade there. I learned to do everything in an abattoir and worked all over a plant, before making my trade as a Slaughterman.

At five am, the chain resumes. The first body comes down the chute. Stunned. There I wait, knife sharp and ready. Make my incision on the left side and, to the right, cut deep. Sever the windpipe. Blood splashes in my face. Wipe it off. The first soul taken for the day for food. Chain shackled around the left hind quarter hock. The labourer pushes the button. The journey begins down the bleed rail along the corridor in the tunnel to bleed out and thrash around.

Knife honed sharp along my steel, ready to do it again. Next, a body drops. Rinse and repeat. All day long. Think of the impact this slowly has on the mind. Commercialised violence, all in the name of food and factory farming. Ok, go organic. The same principles inside an abattoir, just change the labels. Farm fresh, you say. Stand twenty-five metres from the cow at a forty-five-degree angle and aim your rifle between the eyes. One shot. *Bang!* Reload and send a second shot to ensure the kill is made.

Violence is legal for a commercial entity only if production quotas are made and production numbers fill positions.

Often, staff inside these industries come from poor, rural backgrounds. Some have spent time in prison or come from war-torn countries as refugees, from one battleground of losing a family member or a limb to a dictator to another battlefield of survival. I encourage you to watch *Dominion* with a humble heart, and to learn.

One distinct memory stands out and is a trigger to my PTSD. Shadow, a black and white bull calf. One day at an abattoir in Brisbane, I walked into the foetal room where they mine "red gold" or foetal blood from calves for the medical industry. Of all the unborn calves that came down the chute, he stood out to me because he was alive. The labourer grabbed him, measured him up, made two slits into his chest as he was beating and kicking, inserted a tube, and started to pump red gold. His eyes locked onto mine, and I froze. 3, 2, 1 were the blinks, then a lifeless stare into my eyes. This, by far, still haunts me to this day.

I left the beef industry in 2012 due to the physical and mental impact. Journeying through different careers, in 2014 I ended up in transport as a courier where I have been ever since. This became possible due to an inheritance from my father, who helped invest in the industry to get me started. I have had some marginal success with rebuilding a courier franchise territory, and have won incentive trips to Thailand and cash prizes.

MY TURNING POINT

2017 completely changed my direction in life. Here I was, burning out in a dying relationship with an ego so strong from personal development that I did not let anyone in my sphere truly connect with me. In November 2017, I finally broke down and acted out in anger. It was the end of a relationship. I copped an unannounced pregnancy, abortion, and separation in one line, and I didn't take it too well. I didn't act out on my ex. There are no feelings between us now; everything is water under the bridge. But this situation triggered me so badly. I had four dogs under my care and I took my anger out on a sick puppy, killed it, and attempted to hide the evidence by disposing of it in a local river, as I knew bull sharks came through the area. Unfortunately, it didn't go as planned, and the washed-up evidence was found, handed in, and tracked back to me. My house was raided by the RSPCA, all remaining dogs were seized, and my journey to prosecution began.

Research from several very much-argued about historical studies, (such as the *Banduras Bobo* doll experiment), suggests that children who witness or experience aggressive behaviour tend to duplicate it. Other studies, such as *Little Albert* studies, Milgram's *Obedience To Authority*, and Dr Phil Zimbardo's famous *Stanford Prison Experiment*, also suggest this. Other results from these studies also suggest that our environments impact our lives. We see this with second, third, or fourth-generation unemployed families and/or generational criminal behaviour. The "Nature vs. Nurture" argument.

My childhood environment certainly impacted my behaviour and the man I would later become. And how my actions, the result of unsuppressed childhood wounds, would later show up and play out in my life. The evidence certainly suggests this.

On September 20, 2018, I was finally prosecuted after seven months of battling this first case. I pled guilty to one count of "animal cruelty" and two counts of "breach of duty of care." Heavily fined and with two years probation, my circumstances—being thirty-three years of age, this being the first time in front of a magistrate, and being a self-employed courier—and the future impact of a criminal record played in my favour. But I was publicly shamed in the local newspapers and my situation was shared online in different Facebook communities.

On Saturday night, the twenty-first of September, I finished my last shift with a local taxi company as the tidal wave of shaming engulfed my social media and everyone on it. I lost family and friends. It changed a lot of people's perspectives about me. Those I thought were family and good friends disappeared instantly. I lost both my jobs in transport. I lost everything, and my ego came crashing down.

Here I was. I purchased a *.38 Smith and Wesson* pistol from a former courier customer I had known for years, the leader of a local bikie gang at the time. Then I went off to Innisfail in far-north-Queensland to plan my suicide. Far away from the chaos unfolding.

On Monday, I checked into a local Innisfail caravan park. I sat there on Monday night with a loaded 6-shot pistol in my hands. Cocked the hammer back. Put the barrel in my mouth. I could taste the powdery gunpowder residue in my mouth like it had been used. *Click!* went the hammer. It did not discharge. Cocked the hammer a second time. *Click!* went the hammer again. It did not discharge. Cocked the hammer a third time back. Tears streamed down my face. Heavy breathing. Eyes Closed. *Ring! Ring! Ring!* went my phone. I did not want to answer it. I thought it may have been another death threat coming through.

My conscience gave in and I did not discharge the firearm. Instead, I answered my phone to a man I had recently connected with about men's works, and a deep conversation unfolded. This led to an eight-hour phone call, surrender of the weapon, stabilisation and return home, and seeking emergency psychiatric care and suicide watch.

This moment of decision. I could have ignored the call and pulled the trigger. After some conscious thought, I decided to answer the phone and, luckily, I did.

I was introduced to men's support circles which my Probation Officer encouraged along with my regular psychological appointments.

In October I decided to become vegan. I see this as a pathway to start to repay my debt to society and reconnect my head to my heart. Throughout early 2019, I attended some animal rights rallies. I marched in the *March To Close Slaughterhouses* and gave my very first speech on *Poets Corner* in Brisbane. However, my past crept up on me, and I was excluded from the movement.

In October 2018 I got caught with possession of another dog, was formally warned and the dog was seized. I took a relapse in my behaviour. In February 2019 I was caught again with dogs in my possession who were desperate to escape euthanization on kill shelter lists. I thought at the time to repay my debt through compassion unbeknown to the consequences at hand. Wrong!

July 10, 2019, I pled guilty to two counts of "breaching a Prohibition order." Thankfully there were no further charges. They just fined me and I copped a three-month suspended jail sentence over a three-year period. This time wasn't as bad as the State of Origin was on and I had a major distraction to help me deal. Ten days after my case, I was initiated into *The Mankind Project* and undertook my journey of learning to become a responsible man in this world; to make a difference and not damage. This is where I began to learn the tools to give myself a second chance.

I have had a consistent team behind me, holding my feet to the fire. This is no magical unicorn dust-laid path. This path wasn't easy to walk. Change is painful. As men, however, we need to constantly evolve to remain relevant in this world. Being stagnant and comfortable only mentally castrates a man from his potential to become.

You may not have made a mistake as I have. However, my inspiration can somehow have an impact to plant the seeds of progress and change and for you to make a difference in this world.

My lessons have drawn up four pillars of how to give yourself a second chance. Today I share two of these pillars. Change is not easy. Change is painful. This is where the pain, the struggle, and the pressure take—like a piece of coal that goes through seven- hundred-and twenty-five-thousand pounds per inch (five-thousand kilos per centimetre)—to turn into a sparkling diamond. Or buckle and be crushed under that weight. What I offer is a transformation or take a hike. Are you ready to be moulded into something greater? Tony Robbins once said, "When the pain to change exceeds the pain not to change, change will take place."

ACUTE AWARENESS

The first pillar is "Acute Awareness." Awareness is a skill that we men naturally have from our primal days when we had to be consciously aware of our surroundings for survival. Presently, acute awareness is dropping into the moment. Don't deny any feelings. Work out your four main priorities now and see how they are affecting you.

The four priorities are:

1. You

2. Family

3. Work

4. Partner

Men tend to put ourselves last and wonder why we crash. Put them in order currently, and then put them in order of how you think they need to be—with acute awareness.

YOU'RE A MAN: TAKE RESPONSIBILITY

The second pillar is "You're a Man: Take Responsibility." Jocko Willink calls it "Extreme Ownership." Reclaim your balls. Your essence. Fess up! "Yes, this is me. I did that. That was me". Brutal honesty with yourself. Don't apologise to anyone. As a man, you're not sorry. The world isn't sorry for you.

These are two of the four pillars of "How to Give Yourself a Second Chance." Working with me one on one will give you the other two pillars.

Now more than ever, as men the pressures we go through, the confusion, and the constant overwhelm that lead to breakdowns and crisis points can either break us or make us stronger. We need resilience to overcome and learn how to give ourselves a second chance and attempt life once more. When you were born, you cried and the world rejoiced. Live your life so that when you die, the world cries and you rejoice! This is the future of giving yourself a second chance and making a difference in your world and the world around you.

Maybe it is time to give yourself a second chance? Along your journey is it the right time? Each day is a new opportunity to reinvent yourself and make choices that lead towards a more empowering future. Where you can lead by example and make a difference by empowering others along the way. If you're in a male body then I invite you to join me in this journey so that, together, we can create a world with empowered men who are strong in their identity and can lead their role forwards. Because, although life itself is meant to challenge us at the worst of times, our life experiences make us who we are as men. Our current world is screaming out for men to step into their power. To learn the fundamentals at healing themselves which, in turn, has greater impact around them. This means learning to give yourself a second chance, to become stronger and resilient which can help lead to reconnected fathers, and setting a good example to follow. You can do this, can't you? You can, in your current moment of life, right now, give yourself a second chance? Or not...

REFERENCES

Galanaki, E., & Malafantis, K. D. (2022). Albert Bandura's experiments on aggression modeling in children: A psychoanalytic critique. *Frontiers in psychology*, 13, 988877. https://doi.org/10.3389/fpsyg.2022.988877

Mertens G, KrypotosA-M, Engelhard I. (2020) A review on mental imagery in fear conditioning research 100 years since the 'Little Albert' study: *Behaviour Research and Therapy*, Volume 126, 103556, ISSN 0005-7967, https://doi.org/10.1016/j.brat.2020.103556

Bartels, J. M. (2015). The Stanford Prison Experiment in introductory psychology textbooks: *A content analysis. Psychology Learning & Teaching*, 14(1), 36–50. https://doi.org/10.1177/1475725714568007

Griggs, R. A. (2017). Milgram's Obedience Study: *A Contentious Classic Reinterpreted. Teaching of Psychology*, 44(1), 32–37. https://doi.org/10.1177/0098628316677644

ABOUT THE AUTHOR

CRAIG WHITNEY

Craig Whitney is known as the "Second Chance Man." Having been through the justice system himself—four strikes, no prison time; probation with suspended jail sentences—Craig didn't want to be a statistic of the 87.5% recidivism rate in Australia and took advantage of that last opportunity, his second chance, to work with professionals from psychology and criminology to turn his life around.

Equipped with his learnings and life experiences, he now helps men evade that outcome of recidivism by going deeper than the spiritual movement and justice system do. He found the perfect middle.

One of the first men he worked with was serving nine years for armed robbery. After working with Craig, he got his law degree and was called to the bar as a result. That perfect middle!

Based in Brisbane, Craig offers group and 1:1 coaching program on *The 4 Pillars of Giving Yourself a Second Chance* and has a steady following of listeners to his "Last Chance" Podcast.

CONNECT WITH CRAIG HERE:

Website: https://linktr.ee/thesecondchanceman

Free Gift: Free Masterclass on 'How To Give Yourself A Second Chance'

For all socials and link to gift: https://linktr.ee/thesecondchanceman

JOEL D. KENNEDY

BREAKING THE PATTERNS OF FINANCIAL FAILURE

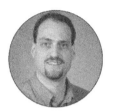

*J*was five-years-old when I was told that my father was never

coming home again.

My family first moved to Alaska when I was too young to remember anything. Just bits and pieces, really. It was like the gold-rush days of commercial fishing, and my dad was drawn to the wild of the Alaskan Gulf Coast, determined to make his fortune trawling the depths for an abundant harvest just below the turbulent waters. But, like many fishermen before and after, he ended his days on earth still searching for the wealth hidden beneath the rolling seas.

Before his final voyage, my dad penned a letter—a prayer, really—asking for help from a God, whom he knew only a little, to protect him from his creditors. I guess his prayer was answered, in a way. He didn't have to worry about that anymore.

Two years later, my mother remarried. I don't blame her for that. I just never understood her choice. Even she admits she didn't love him, at least not at first. My mom was supposedly directed by God to marry him and when she confessed that she didn't have any feelings for him, as the story

135

goes, she was suddenly given a deep love for him which she took as a sign.

We were often reminded of this story as if it was some kind of miracle but, to me, it just seemed like justification—maybe because it was usually brought up after they had a big fight.

Growing up, my mom and stepdad fought a lot. Even when they weren't arguing, there was a tension that never really went away. Things would seem fine on the surface, but my sister and I were always wary, trying to avoid whatever the unknowable thing was that would set my step-dad off and incite a reaction from my mom that would turn a fun family outing into a raging inferno of vitriol.

As I recall, their arguments were almost always about money. Even if that wasn't the main topic, it was like that was the source of the underlying tension—the tinder waiting for a spark. In time, I would come to understand that the cloud we were living under was fear. The fear of running out of money was ever-present.

We weren't poor, per se. We were what some would call lower-middle-class. My mother was frugal with the food budget, mostly buying things that were "on sale," and at times we had to use food stamps (back when they were actual stamps) but as far as I recall, we never went hungry.

In the tiny fishing village where we lived before my dad passed, we would have actually been considered the "rich" family. We owned the largest fishing boat as well as the local general store, which my mom managed while my dad was out fishing, and we had our own private plane. But my parents also had a lot of debt.

Fortuitously, my dad had taken out two life insurance policies, one for $250,000 and one for $1,000,000. Unfortunately, he had let the latter lapse just a couple of months before he died—probably due to lack of money to cover the premiums—just past the grace period. While a quarter-of-a-million dollars seemed like a lot of money in the 1980s, I often wonder how things would have been different if that larger policy was still in force.

My mom moved us to Juneau, the closest "big city," where she bought a modest home in a trailer park. By the time all the debts were paid off, the money from that smaller policy was pretty much gone. She got a job and put us in school, but we were just barely getting by. It certainly wasn't easy for a single mom with three kids and no other family around to help.

I wouldn't be surprised if the prospect of a steady salary and government pension was perhaps more of a factor in her decision to marry than she would admit.

Just a short time into their marriage, my step-dad abruptly quit his government job in a heated disagreement with his boss, and decided to go into business for himself. I guess he figured the freedom of being your own boss was better than the security of a steady paycheck.

Between my dad and stepdad, I guess you could say the idea of working for yourself had been pretty well planted in me. By the age of seventeen, I had already started my first business—fixing small engines and sharpening chainsaws. That was the beginning of my own tenuous relationship with money.

Fast-forward about twenty years to find me college-educated, married with kids, good job, house (mortgage), nice cars (payments), credit cards (maxed)... The whole works.

Happy? Not really.

Over time, I developed chronic, unexplained health issues, lost my job, house, cars, and ended up filing for bankruptcy.

Fast-forward another ten years and we were living on an island in the northwest corner of Washington State, having all but recovered from our previous financial problems. I had launched a tech support business that was growing, and our life was getting back on track.

Yet we could never figure out why we always seemed to be scraping the bottom of the barrel. Month after month. Year after year. Decade after decade. We would get close to where we felt, "This is it! We're on the right path to being financially stable." And then something would happen that would take the wind out of our sails.

We never seemed to have a chance to save much money before something happened. An unexpected expense would pop up, a health issue, career change, house move, or a premature baby (we had a couple of those). Almost like playing a real-time, expanded version of Milton Bradley's *The Game of Life*.

Remember that game? Spin the wheel and see what fate has to offer you. You choose whether to go to college (by going into debt) or start a career. Much of that game seems so random—just like *real* life, I guess.

In 2015, my wife left her job to work with me and help grow our business. It felt great to be working for myself again, and loving it. I still had chronic health issues, but I was managing them. I also loved that we were able to bring the kids in and teach them how to fix computers and run a company. We were feeling good, spinning that wheel, and gleefully moving our maxed-out minivan forward on the game board.

Then we landed on that dreaded space. You know, the one where the landlord knocks on your door and tells you that you have thirty days to move out? Yeah, that one.

"No problem," we thought. "We'll just find another place. Maybe we're even in a position to buy a house and start putting down roots." So we started to look for just the right house for our growing family. We applied with rental agencies and mortgage companies, just to cover all of our bases. And we kept looking... And applying... And looking... And applying...

It didn't take long before we realized that in the area we lived, near Seattle, there was a housing supply shortage and market prices had been going up steadily since the crash of 2008. And with eight kids, two dogs, and my mother-in-law living with us at that time, our options were even more limited, so our monthly housing costs would be going up—by a lot!

By the time we found a place, we were paying more than double the amount we had been paying just a few months earlier. Imagine having to suddenly come up with an additional $1500 per month out of an already tight budget. Besides being only a temporary arrangement, the truth was that we really couldn't afford it. But at the time, we had little choice.

After about a year of searching and bouncing our family from one temporary situation to another, we finally faced the reality that we had to move back to the mainland. To make matters worse, we couldn't find a buyer for the business and were forced to close it down. We were devastated. All of those dreams and plans we had made, and we just had to walk away.

But, being the eternal optimists that we are, it didn't keep us down for long. With the help of our friends, family, and even some of our former customers, we were able to afford to rent a house in a thriving area just a couple of hours north, near the Canadian border. It wasn't ideal, but once we got established up there, we felt we could be in a position to buy it and make some improvements.

Spin the wheel. Move the marker. *Tap, tap, tap.* Rent goes up another thirty percent. And here we go again. Spin after spin. Setback after setback.

Within the course of a year, we were literally homeless—living in cars and tents that friends gave us. Thankfully, it was summertime and we always found a way to make lemonade out of lemons, as they say. We thought, "You know, people spend thousands of dollars to go camping every year. Why not enjoy it?"

Determined to make the best of it, we decided that, no matter the situation, we would be grateful for all the blessings we had, as well as for those that had not yet materialized. In doing so, we had begun to understand what true abundance really is.

Even so, we felt like we still couldn't quite get a handle on our finances. It's like we were living in abundance in every area of our life, except money. It was clear that we needed to re-evaluate our relationship with money. But where to start?

Everyone has a relationship with money. I know we tend to think of money as this impersonal, soulless thing that we all strive for but are never supposed to care for, right? If you *do* love money, that's usually considered bad, especially in conservative Christian homes like the one I grew up in. We were taught that the love of money is the root of all evil. So, the idea of having a relationship with it was almost sacrilege.

As we look deeper, it can be surprising just how much our relationship with money is tied to our relationships with people, especially the people we trust the most. The people who have taught us, people who mentored us and gave us our financial foundation—that's where our relationship with money starts. But it's not where it has to end.

It was decades before I finally faced the one relationship that was holding me back from financial success: my parents.

Now, you might be thinking, "Oh, here we go. Another sob story about how someone's parents did them wrong." But here's the thing—if we're not willing to look back and assess our past truthfully, then we will always be stuck repeating the same mistakes that we, and our parents, and their parents, have made time after time, generation after generation.

As the saying goes, those who don't face their past are destined to repeat it. I finally came to realize that if I didn't face my past and address those things that were causing me to repeat the same behaviors over and over, I was just going to keep doing the same things, over and over. And I was never going to get out of this cycle.

My relationship with my parents has had its ups and downs and, as I looked back, I could finally start to see how our financial life was mirroring this same pattern. But no matter how many "up" times there were, the long-term trend was definitely down.

Not long ago, something happened that finally woke me up to this fact.

When we were first getting started in the financial industry, I was talking with my stepdad about the business. While finances can often be a touchy subject for people, we had discussed money matters before, so I thought we were having a rational conversation. Boy, was I wrong! Without warning, he started questioning our judgment, motives and integrity.

By this time, I was fairly accustomed to his sudden flare-ups, and I could have treated this one like we had the others in years past, just to placate him. But this time was different. I realized that if I didn't do something different this time then nothing was ever going to change.

And change was exactly what we needed right then. Drastic change. Life-altering change.

Then I did the one thing that changed my relationship with money forever. I took a cold, hard look at my parents' financial situation and asked myself, "Is this where I want to be in thirty years? Do I really want to live my entire life under the cloud of fear that we're going to run out of money?"

In that moment, it became clear to me that unless this was the future I wanted for myself, my wife, and my family, it was time for us to go in a completely different direction. Even if that meant severing the relationship with my step-dad. So I did just that.

"Clank!" (That's the sound of train tracks switching, in case you didn't catch that.)

As soon as I made the decision to disconnect and stop emulating my parents' financial life, our financial outlook started changing. The change didn't happen instantly, mind you. Just like it takes a little while for an entire train to switch over to another track, it's going to take time for our lives to manifest the change. But we knew right away that something was different!

It's freeing to know you don't have to do things the way your parents did them.

I'm not saying you need to completely cut ties with them. Nor am I saying that you need to reject everything they have taught you. But if it's clear that that relationship is not healthy for you, it's probably not healthy for them either and it might be time to part ways, especially if you can identify a similar pattern match in their lives and in yours. And it doesn't have to be your parents, either.

In every relationship, there can be a lot of tension centered around money. In fact, I would say that money is the number one point of contention in most marriages or domestic partnerships. But it's not so much about the money itself as it is about how people treat their money. And how people treat money directly correlates with how they treat each other.

Sometimes our finances affect our relationships, and sometimes our relationships affect our finances. It can be both, and often has lasting ripple effects.

My wife's financial upbringing was a bit different from mine, although she also felt a lot of tension around the topic of money. Her dad made most of the financial decisions and her mom was rarely included in those decisions. Consequently, when their marriage finally ended in divorce (due largely to lack of trust), her mom knew little about how to manage her own finances.

But the effects of that relationship didn't stop there. Some of those mindsets were passed down to my wife so, early in our marriage, her tendency was to leave financial decisions to me. Every couple has to figure out their roles along the way, and money plays a significant part in that. When we started homeschooling the kids, for example, one of us needed to stay home with the kids. This created some financial strain, but we both agreed it was worth the sacrifice.

Over the years we switched roles multiple times, which gave us valuable perspective as both breadwinner and homemaker and made it easier to talk about money. And while we have always had a strong marriage, we were still kind of stuck in the "money is bad" mindset. Not that we were afraid of money, it was more like we were afraid to get too comfortable with it.

It wasn't until we worked with people in the financial industry that we really began to see this, and that's when our financial life started to really shift. But just wanting to be better with money wasn't enough; we had to start cultivating relationships with people who were good with money and who still shared our values. So we did just that!

Now, we're teaching others to better understand money and how to start building real wealth—even if, like us, they're not getting started until later in life. We are so blessed to be a part of a company that is built on the foundation of helping people from all backgrounds to be financially successful, no matter who they are, where they come from, or what their net worth is.

WHAT IS YOUR RELATIONSHIP WITH MONEY?

You might be one of those people who just treat money as a necessary evil, like we did. Or you might be obsessed with money to the point that it turns other people off. Maybe you just try to ignore money matters as much as possible, and then blame others for your financial problems.

You might need to ask yourself, "Are my relationships suffering because I'm neglecting my relationship with money?" If you're ready to see a dramatic change in your financial situation, here are some things you can work on right now.

#1: Focus on improving your relationship with money

First, you have to be honest with yourself. Ask some hard questions:

Does money stress me out? Or, do I obsess about it?

Do I avoid the topic or procrastinate looking at my finances?

Do I spend without thinking about where the money is coming from?

What can I do, right now, to change that?

As you do this, you will likely find that just making more money is not the solution to your financial problems. Yes, it can help in the near-term, but if you step back and look at the bigger picture, you might find that your mindsets are the real problem. For example, if you don't feel you deserve money, then that is what you will manifest in your life. Time to change those mindsets that aren't serving you.

#2: Acknowledge that it's not too late to change course

If your long-term trend is in a downward spiral, like ours was, it's time for a drastic change. Don't be afraid to reevaluate the relationships in your life that have had the most profound effect on your financial health, and to prune the ones that are taking you in the wrong direction. Even if you are no longer in that relationship, you could still be holding on to some residual ideas or mindsets. It might be time to let them go.

#3: *Develop new relationships that will help you change and stay that course*

As you recognize unhealthy relationships in your life, begin to replace them with ones that serve you better—people who are going in the direction you want to go. Don't just try to cozy up to the next rich person you see. Find people with a solid wealth-building mindset and character that you want to emulate in your life. Look for people who have money, who are not afraid to work hard, but who can also enjoy life and get along with people.

I promise you that doing these three things will have a dramatic effect on your life, and not just financially. But that's only the beginning. When you're ready to start building real wealth, send me a message via the email address listed in my bio. Tell me a little about how this chapter helped you, and in return, I'll send you a special gift that will help you get your financial life on track to experiencing true abundance.

Remember that living in abundance isn't just about having a lot of money; it's about being grateful for what you have and for what you don't *yet* have. It starts by recognizing that there is plenty to go around. So much of the financial world around us is based on a mindset of scarcity. That's when greed and fear start to take over. Only when we understand that there is more than enough for all of us will we truly begin living in abundance.

ABOUT THE AUTHOR

JOEL D. KENNEDY

As a full-time homeschooling dad, licensed financial professional, educator and documentary filmmaker, Joel D. Kennedy has never shied away from a challenge. Raised in Alaska, he learned from a young age how to survive in the wilderness and build a cabin from scratch, but he was never taught how to build wealth or survive a financial crisis.

After spending decades trying to free himself from ghosts of failures past, Joel had all but resigned himself to a life of financial scarcity. It wasn't until he was in his forties that he finally confronted the one thing holding him back from experiencing financial abundance.

Today he and his wife, Bethany, are living the life of their dreams, traveling the country in an RV with their kids while helping families and individuals get on track financially and learn how to live a life of true abundance.

CONNECT WITH JOEL HERE:

Website: https://TrueAbundance.us

Free Gift: For a free session, email: Book@TrueAbundance.us

For all socials: https://linktr.ee/JoelDKennedy

ABOUT YOUR WORDS HAVE POWER

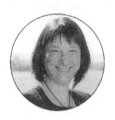

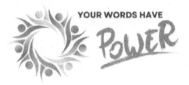

*T*he inspiration to create this book came out of *Your Words*
Have Power (YWHP), a multi-platform organisation founded by Wendy
Corner. YWHP is committed to helping speakers who seek to share their
messages and stories on a global scale to inspire people to live their lives
more fully.

It is their mission to challenge the hearts and minds of their audiences by
creating an indelible imprint on humanity, forever raising the vibration
of human consciousness by poking the bear, by being our unique selves,
and by not accepting the status quo! When we share our stories and
speak our message, we are recognised for our own unique qualities.

Wendy Corner realised that there are many passionate speakers
eager to make a difference and get their message out there, but without
any knowledge of how to reach those bigger stages. In 2022, she
designed YWHP to bridge this gap.

Today, YWHP offers virtual and physical stages for speakers to test and spread their message. It offers coaching programmes as well as different avenues (including book projects and live events) for speakers to challenge the hearts and minds of their intended audience.

With her thirty-years' experience as a Speech Pathologist, TEDx Trainer since 2018, and Speaker Coach to business and community leaders around the world, Wendy leads the way in making a difference and has created a dynamic community to do just that.

Wendy helps aspiring and seasoned speakers create a strategy and plan to get their message out across multiple platforms, and guides her clients to refine that message and improve their craft in ways that help their stories to make a bigger impact.

In 2022, eighty-nine speakers tested their message on the YWHP platform and grew our audience to 6000+ followers. They became prolific speakers and were able to profoundly impact their audiences within their ten-minute presentations. Most of them realised the impact they could make as they saw more people gravitate towards their message.

The theme of 2023 became M.A.D.: a year for Making A Difference. Hence, we have created this book and the M.A.D. Summit will follow in early 2024.

If you are an aspiring author and speaker looking to make a bigger impact, increase your authority and gain global reach, then reach out to Wendy to join the second edition of our M.A.D. book series: Ways to Magnify Abundance, Vitality & Freedom.

CONNECT WITH *YOUR WORDS HAVE POWER* AND WENDY HERE:

Website: https://www.ywhp.events

For all socials: https//linkgtr.ee/commcoach

ABOUT SPARKBIZOPS

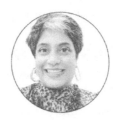

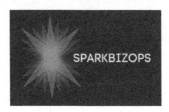

$\mathcal{S}$ PARKBIZOPS, the brainchild of Jenny Vaz, operates on a

mission to help business owners create and manifest the best ideas for their clients and employees.

In Making A Difference, SparkBizOps took care of the book launch marketing campaign and social media outreach.

Founded in 2021, they have since partnered with businesses from the US, Zimbabwe, Australia, and Canada expand their business in the digital and global world, as well as co-develop ideas that change the world for the better!

Their work has taken the organisation across multiple sectors: creative agencies, publishing, life coaching, sustainability consulting, female-led startups, and martial arts gyms. Clients have sought their expertise in the areas of business strategy, market research, white paper authoring (successful bid for USD 20m fund), content creation and delivery including social media and website, and creative designs, as well as payment automations, business process design, and data and analytics.

As the founder of SparkBizOps, Jenny helps entrepreneurs across the world clean up bottlenecks and broken processes, proposing and implementing strategies to direct more of their energy, time and resources in their business and teams towards their zones of genius.

She is an international bestselling author and speaker who attributes all her success in her life and professional career to focusing on her innate strengths and her ability to add value to any opportunity that's been presented to her. This talent, coupled with drive and relentlessness, has taken her around the world to live and work in seven different countries across four continents.

For over twenty years, Jenny has worked as a technology consultant and strategist with government and billion-dollar businesses right down to solo operators. Her unique skillset zooms in on her client's expertise and unique value proposition that centers on the heart of the person in front of her and helps them realise how truly powerful they, and their business, are.

Jenny's clients choose to work with her because SparkBizOps operate like an extension of their business, going the extra mile, and treating it with the same care as they treat their own. They will co-create your strategy and do all the heavy-lifting implementation so that you and your team can focus more on your zones of genius and take greater care of your clients and employees.

CONNECT WITH JENNY HERE:

Website: www.sparkbizops.io

For socials and all other links: linktr.ee/jennyvaz

ABOUT HILLE HOUSE PUBLISHING

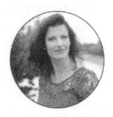

$\mathcal{K}$RYSTAL HILLE founded Hille House Publishing in early 2021 in answer to the call of collaborating with thought leaders so that, collectively, we can raise the vibration of the planet, one person, one story and one book at a time, bringing humanity to a tipping point of personal power, deeper connection, and sovereignty.

With this eighth anthology, we have now helped over 200 thought leaders from twenty-six countries and six continents to become international bestselling authors, share their stories, and position themselves as leading experts on a global stage alongside the likes of lead authors like Dr. John Demartini, Dr. Larry Farwell, and Lorie Ladd, whom we've attracted into our books.

We aim to continue creating books that awaken, inspire, and empower the reader into deeper sovereignty and connection. If you are passionate about this as well, we would love to hear from you.

Whether you are an individual ready to publish your finished manuscript or interested in contributing to one of our collaborative books, or you are the head of an organisation seeking to showcase your members, clients, or students, to create greater brand awareness and exposure, we welcome you. Alternatively, you may be ready to write your own book but don't want to do it alone. In that case, we offer group writing containers where you can collaborate with others.

As Hille House Publishing's founder, Krystal has known since her teens that she was here to help humanity in some way. Her methods have evolved with her across three professional sectors: theatre, personal development, and publishing.

One thing has remained consistent, her intuitive ability to 'see people' in ways that they may not have seen themselves and her passion for empowering- and bringing the best out in people. First, as a theatre director, where she married the innate essence and highest potential of her actors with that of the character so they could create powerful stage performances.

Then, in her thirties, she trained as a transformational coach, Reiki Master, NLP practitioner and Tantra Teacher, helping clients live their best life, especially women who were looking to reconnect with their embodied, feminine essence, harmonise discipline with flow, and step into their soul leadership.

Now, in her late forties, Krystal has come full circle, returning to her love for literature that has been alive since her childhood and led her to become the editor of her school magazine and awarded her a distinction in her BA Hons in English Literature and Theatre Studies.

She now enjoys guiding change makers and conscious creatives through the transformational journey of becoming published authors and writing their best books or chapter, so that their passion can ignite global change.

With 30 years in leadership, a background in theatre directing, and female empowerment, Krystal is a multiple international #1 bestselling author, winner of the CREA Brainz Global Business Award 2021. Aware of her multidimensional self, pre-Covid, Krystal co-facilitated spiritual retreats to Egypt and ran the Temple Nights across Australia.

She is a popular contributor to international festivals, summits, and podcasts and has co-written two solo books and contributed to further five anthologies with another solo book in the making.

Originally from Germany, Krystal lives with her two pre-teen children in county Victoria, Australia.

We would love to hear from you if you would like to join future multi-author books, create a compilation book for your organisation, publish or write your solo book through Hille House Publishing.

CONNECT WITH KRYSTAL HERE:

Website: https://hillehousepublishing.com

Email: krystal@krystalhille.com

Socials and more: https://linktr.ee/krystalhille

Made in the USA
Las Vegas, NV
20 August 2023

76363163R00100